Equine Infectious Diseases

Editor

BRETT A. SPONSELLER

VETERINARY CLINICS OF NORTH AMERICA: EQUINE PRACTICE

www.vetequine.theclinics.com

Consulting Editor
RAMIRO E. TORIBIO

April 2023 • Volume 39 • Number 1

ELSEVIER

1600 John F. Kennedy Boulevard • Suite 1800 • Philadelphia, Pennsylvania, 19103-2899

http://www.vetequine.theclinics.com

VETERINARY CLINICS OF NORTH AMERICA: EQUINE PRACTICE Volume 39, Number 1
April 2023 ISSN 0749-0739, ISBN-13: 978-0-323-96063-2

Editor: Taylor Hayes
Developmental Editor: Ann Gielou Posedio

Veterinary Clinics of North America: Equine Practice (ISSN 0749-0739) is published in April, August, and December by Elsevier Inc., 360 Park Avenue South, New York, NY 10010-1710. Business and Editorial Offices: 1600 John F. Kennedy Blvd., Suite 1800, Philadelphia, PA 19103-2899. Subscription prices are $308.00 per year (domestic individuals), $647.00 per year (domestic institutions), $100.00 per year (domestic students/residents), $351.00 per year (Canadian individuals), $814.00 per year (Canadian institutions), $383.00 per year (international individuals), $814.00 per year (international institutions), $100.00 per year (Canadian students/residents), and $180.00 per year (international students/residents). To receive student/resident rate, orders must be accompanied by name of affiliated institution, date of term, and the signature of program/residency coordinator on institution letterhead. Orders will be billed at individual rate until proof of status is received. Foreign air speed delivery is included in all *Clinics* subscription prices. All prices are subject to change without notice. **POSTMASTER:** Send address changes to *Veterinary Clinics of North America: Equine Practice*, 3251 Riverport Lane, Maryland Heights, MO 63043. Customer Service (orders, claims, online, change of address): Elsevier Health Sciences Division, Subscription **Customer Service, 3251 Riverport Lane, Maryland Heights, MO 63043. Tel: 1-800-654-2452 (U.S. and Canada); 314-447-8871 (outside U.S. and Canada). Fax: 314-447-8029. E-mail: journalscustomerservice-usa@elsevier.com (for print support);** E-mail: **journalsonlinesupport-usa@elsevier.com (for online support).**

Reprints. For copies of 100 or more of articles in this publication, please contact the Commercial Reprints Department, Elsevier Inc., 360 Park Avenue South, New York, NY 10010-1710. Tel.: 212-633-3874; Fax: 212-633-3820; E-mail: reprints@elsevier.com.

Veterinary Clinics of North America: Equine Practice is covered in *MEDLINE/PubMed (Index Medicus), Excerpta Medica, Current Contents/Agriculture, Biology and Environmental Sciences,* and *ISI.*

Contributors

CONSULTING EDITOR

RAMIRO E. TORIBIO, DVM, MS, PhD
Diplomate, American College of Veterinary Internal Medicine; Professor and Trueman
Endowed Chair of Equine Medicine and Surgery, College of Veterinary Medicine, The Ohio
State University, Columbus, Ohio, USA

EDITOR

BRETT A. SPONSELLER, DVM, PhD
Diplomate, American College of Veterinary Internal Medicine; Associate Professor,
Departments of Veterinary Microbiology and Preventive Medicine and Veterinary Clinical
Sciences, College of Veterinary Medicine, Iowa State University, Ames, Iowa, USA

AUTHORS

ASHLEY G. BOYLE, DVM
Diplomate, American College of Veterinary Internal Medicine - Large Animal; Associate
Professor, Department of Clinical Studies, New Bolton Center, University of Pennsylvania,
School of Veterinary Medicine, Kennett Square, Pennsylvania, USA

BRANDY A. BURGESS, DVM, MSc, PhD
Diplomate, American College of Veterinary Internal Medicine (Large Animal Internal
Medicine); Diplomate, American College of Veterinary Preventive Medicine; Associate
Professor, Department of Population Health, College of Veterinary Medicine, University of
Georgia, Athens, Georgia, USA

FRANCISCO O. CONRADO, DVM, MSc
Diplomate, American College of Veterinary Pathologists; Assistant Professor of Clinical
Pathology, Department of Comparative Pathobiology, Tufts University, Cummings School
of Veterinary Medicine, Hospital for Large Animals, North Grafton, Massachusetts, USA

JENNIFER G. JANES, DVM, PhD
Diplomate, American College of Veterinary Pathologists; Associate Professor, Department
of Veterinary Science, University of Kentucky, Veterinary Diagnostic Laboratory,
Lexington, Kentucky, USA

JAMIE J. KOPPER, DVM, PhD
Diplomate, American College of Veterinary Internal Medicine - Large Animal Internal
Medicine; Diplomate, American College of Veterinary Emergency and Critical Care - Large
Animal; Iowa State University, College of Veterinary Medicine, Ames, Iowa, USA

DEEPA ASHWARYA KUTTAPPAN, BVSc, AH, MVSc, PhD, DABT
Study Director, Toxicology Laboratory Corporation of America, Indianapolis, Indiana, USA

DANIELA LUETHY, DVM, MPH
Diplomate, American College of Veterinary Internal Medicine; Clinical Assistant Professor, Large Animal Internal Medicine, Large Animal Clinical Sciences, College of Veterinary Medicine, University of Florida, Gainesville, Florida, USA

SHANKUMAR MOOYOTTU, BVSc, MVSc, MS, PhD
Diplomate, American College of Veterinary Pathologists; Associate Professor of Pathology, Department of Pathobiology, College of Veterinary Medicine, Auburn University, Auburn, Alabama, USA

ROSE NOLEN-WALSTON, DVM
Diplomate, American College of Veterinary Internal Medicine; Associate Professor of Internal Medicine, Department of Clinical Studies, University of Pennsylvania, New Bolton Center, Pennsylvania, USA

ANDREA OLIVER, DVM
Department of Clinical Studies, University of Pennsylvania, New Bolton Center, Kennett Square, Pennsylvania, USA

ANGELA M. PELZEL-MCCLUSKEY, DVM, MS
Equine Epidemiologist, United States Department of Agriculture, Animal and Plant Health Inspection Service, Veterinary Services, Fort Collins, Colorado, USA

NICOLA PUSTERLA, DVM, PhD
Department of Medicine and Epidemiology, School of Veterinary Medicine, University of California, Davis, Davis, California, USA

REBECCA E. RUBY, MSc, BVSc
Diplomate, American College of Veterinary Pathologists; Diplomate, American College of Veterinary Internal Medicine - Large Animal Internal Medicine; Assistant Professor, Department of Veterinary Science, University of Kentucky, Veterinary Diagnostic Laboratory, Lexington, Kentucky, USA

MACARENA G. SANZ, DVM, MS, PhD
Diplomate, American College of Veterinary Internal Medicine-Large Animal; Associate Professor Equine Medicine, Washington State University, Pullman, Washington, USA

BRETT A. SPONSELLER, DVM, PhD
Diplomate, American College of Veterinary Internal Medicine; Associate Professor, Departments of Veterinary Microbiology and Preventive Medicine and Veterinary Clinical Sciences, College of Veterinary Medicine, Iowa State University, Ames, Iowa, USA

ALLISON J. STEWART, BVSc (Hons I), MS, PhD, MANZCVS
Diplomate, American College of Veterinary Internal Medicine; Diplomate, American College of Veterinary Emergency Critical Care; UQ VETS Equine Specialist Hospital, School of Veterinary Science, University of Queensland, Gatton, Queensland, Australia

SANDRA D. TAYLOR, DVM, PhD
Associate Professor, Department of Veterinary Clinical Sciences, College of Veterinary Medicine, Purdue University, West Lafayette, Indiana, USA

XUELI WANG, DVM
UQ VETS Equine Specialist Hospital, School of Veterinary Science, University of Queensland, Gatton, Queensland, Australia

JESSICA C. WISE, BVetBio/BVSc, MANZCVS, DVStud
Diplomate, European College of Equine Internal Medicine; UQ VETS Equine Specialist Hospital, School of Veterinary Science, University of Queensland, Gatton, Queensland, Australia

Contents

Neorickettsia risticii. However, N. findlayensis has been isolated from affected horses. Horses typically become infected upon ingestion of Neorickettsia spp.-infected trematodes within aquatic insects. The most common clinical signs include diarrhea, fever, anorexia, lethargy and colic. The diagnostic test of choice for PHF is PCR of blood and feces. Tetracyclines remain an effective treatment. Supportive care, including fluid therapy, colloid administration, NSAID and anti-endotoxin medication, and digital cryotherapy, is also necessary in some cases.

Equine rotavirus is one of the most common causes of infectious diarrhea in foals. Although the infection itself is self-limiting, the resulting diarrhea is due to multiple mechanisms and can be severe, requiring supportive care including fluid and electrolyte support. Prompt diagnosis is important for treatment and biosecurity decisions and can be achieved by several means. Prevention, while imperfect, currently relies on vaccination of pregnant mares before parturition, ingestion of adequate colostrum from vaccinated mares and biosecurity measures.

Coronaviruses are a group of related RNA viruses that cause diseases in mammals and birds. In equids, equine coronavirus has been associated with diarrhea in foals and lethargy, fever, anorexia, and occasional gastrointestinal signs in adult horses. Although horses seem to be susceptible to the human severe acute respiratory syndrome coronavirus-2 (SARS-CoV-2) based on the high homology to the ACE-2 receptor, they seem to be incidental hosts because of occasional SARS-CoV-2 spillover from humans. However, until more clinical and seroepidemiological data are available, it remains important to monitor equids for possible transmission from humans with clinical or asymptomatic COVID-19.

A variety of infectious agents including viral, bacterial, and fungal organisms can cause equine abortion and placentitis. Knowledge of normal anatomy and the common pattern distribution of different infectious agents will assist the practitioner in evaluating the fetus and/or placenta, collecting appropriate samples for further testing, and in some cases, forming a presumptive diagnosis. In all cases, it is recommended to confirm the diagnosis with molecular, serologic, or microbiological testing. If a causative agent can be identified, then appropriate biosecurity and vaccination measures can be instituted on the farm.

Vesicular stomatitis (VS) is a vector-borne livestock disease caused by vesicular stomatitis New Jersey virus (VSNJV) or vesicular stomatitis Indiana virus (VSIV). The disease circulates endemically in northern South America, Central America, and Mexico and only occasionally causes outbreaks in the United States. Over the past 20 years, VS outbreaks in the southwestern and Rocky Mountain regions occurred periodically with incursion years followed by virus overwintering and subsequent expansion outbreak years. The regulatory response by animal health officials prevents the spread of disease by animals with lesions and manages trade impacts. Recent US outbreaks highlight potential climate change impacts on insect vectors or other transmission-related variables.

VETERINARY CLINICS OF NORTH AMERICA: EQUINE PRACTICE

SERIES OF RELATED INTEREST

Veterinary Clinics of North America: Food Animal Practice
https://www.vetfood.theclinics.com/

THE CLINICS ARE NOW AVAILABLE ONLINE!
Access your subscription at:
www.theclinics.com

Preface

Getting Prepared

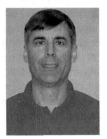

Brett A. Sponseller, DVM, PhD
Editor

One constant in veterinary practice is "change," and in the case of infectious diseases, not only is our understanding of potential pathogens improving—a positive change— but also many features of the pathogens are changing, perhaps posing new clinical challenges. Antimicrobial resistance is an increasingly concerning feature in managing bacterial diseases in horses of all ages, including *Rhodococcus equi*. Dr Sanz provides context for management options, including active surveillance, and reviews considerations in adjunct plasma administration. As for *Clostridioides difficile*, a contentious name change has been made, and the recent detection of "human isolates" in companion animals has raised the possibility of (reverse) zoonotic transmission of *C difficile*, emphasizing the need for a One Health approach in equine practice. Drs Kuttappan, Mooyottu, and Sponseller summarize disease associated with *C difficile* and review recent findings spanning several equine enteric clostridial diseases. Dr Burgess provides a complete synopsis of *Salmonella* from the standpoint of clinical disease, shedding, risk factors, mitigation approaches, and public health concerns, while Dr Taylor reviews the known causative agents of Potomac Horse Fever and treatment approaches, and Dr Kopper reviews rotaviral diarrhea, providing an update on a ruminant-like group B rotavirus outbreak that appeared in 2022 in central Kentucky. Another RNA virus, also prone to change, is the fodder of Dr Pusterla's exposé and pertains to equine coronavirus; however, he provides a word of caution regarding SARS-2 and the potential for adaptation to the equine host. Drs Ruby and Janes review infectious causes of equine placentitis and abortion and provide helpful suggestions to optimize obtaining a diagnosis. Drs Stewart, Wang, and Wise review another RNA virus causing high mortality in horses and having zoonotic potential, Hendra virus, and the very real threat it poses to humans and other outdoor animals. Dr Luethy provides a complete overview of the clinical and public health considerations of the main encephalomyelitis-causing arboviruses (Eastern equine encephalitis virus [EEE], Western equine encephalitis virus [WEE], Venezuelan equine encephalitis virus [VEE], and

Vet Clin Equine 39 (2023) xiii–xiv
https://doi.org/10.1016/j.cveq.2022.12.001
0749-0739/23/© 2022 Published by Elsevier Inc.

West Nile virus [WNV]) affecting horses, and in some cases, humans. Dr Boyle summarizes the past 10 years of advances in managing *Streptococcus equi* subspecies *equi* infection with an emphasis on containing spread. Drs Oliver, Conrado, and Nolen-Walston review Equine Granulocytic Anaplasmosis, a disease well characterized in horses in 1969 and then in humans 25 years later, necessitating an eventual name change of the pathogen from *Ehrlicia equi* to *Anaplasma phagocytophilum*. Dr Pelzel-McCluskey reminds us of the equine practitioner's role in containing spread of Vesicular Stomatitis Virus (VSV), another RNA virus that is also an arbovirus. The recent northward incursion of VSV suggests a possible expansion of the range of the vector or vectors within the United States. In sum, the clinical landscape of equine infectious diseases is ever evolving, requiring an updated awareness of the field.

One of the earliest infectious disease experts, Louis Pasteur, stated that, "in the fields of observation, chance favors only the prepared mind." I very much appreciate the expertise and effort these authors put forth to better prepare us for another day of clinical observation.

Brett A. Sponseller, DVM, PhD
Departments of Veterinary Microbiology &
Preventive Medicine and Veterinary Clinical Sciences
College of Veterinary Medicine
Iowa State University
1809 South Riverside Drive
Ames, IA 50011-3619, USA

E-mail address:
baspon@iastate.edu

Rhodococcus equi–What is New This Decade?

Macarena G. Sanz, DVM, MS, PhD, DACVIM-LA

KEYWORDS

- *Rhodococcus equi* • Pneumonia • Hyperimmune plasma • Antimicrobial resistance
- Foal

KEY POINTS

- Foals are infected with *Rhodococcus equi* shortly after birth.
- Many infected foals develop self-resolving subclinical disease.
- Treatment of subclinical disease has led to the development of antimicrobial-resistant strains.
- Administration of hyperimmune plasma minimizes the severity of pneumonia but does not prevent infection.
- Better biomarkers are needed to aid targeted treatment and minimize the development of resistance to antimicrobials.
- Questions remain regarding prophylactic strategies against this pathogen.

Our understanding of *R equi* pathogenesis has changed over the last decade, and this knowledge has translated to a new set of recommendations regarding prophylaxis, treatment, and diagnosis. Before thoracic ultrasonography became widely available, it was proposed that foals became infected with *R equi* around 3 to 6 month of age, the period of time when the clinical signs were observed. With the introduction of thoracic ultrasonography as a screening tool, it became apparent that foals were infected early in life and disease progressed slowly until the development of clinical signs months after the initial infection. Unfortunately, early diagnosis of infection was also associated with an increased rate of treatment of subclinical foals and rapid selection of antimicrobial resistant (AMR) strains of *R equi*. The goal of this article is to provide the equine practitioner with a useful summary of the current recommendations that are supported by new literature and to highlight the areas that require further investigation.

RHODOCOCCUS EQUI IN FOALS

Rhodococcus equi (*R equi*) remains the most common cause of subacute or chronic granulomatous bronchopneumonia in foals less than 5 months of age.[1,2] This disease

Washington State University, Pullman, WA, USA
E-mail address: macarena@wsu.edu

Vet Clin Equine 39 (2023) 1–14
https://doi.org/10.1016/j.cveq.2022.11.002
vetequine.theclinics.com

continues to have a major financial impact on the horse industry due to the cost and labor associated with treatment and prevention strategies and the lack of a commercial vaccine.

R equi is a gram-positive intracellular bacterial pathogen that is normally present in the environment and in the manure of healthy herbivores.[3] Under breeding farm situations, the environmental concentration of *R equi* increases because the organism replicates in horse manure and infected foals shed larger amounts of virulent *R equi* in their feces.[4] Conditions that favor aerosolization of *R equi* such as high foal density and hot dry weather have been recognized as risk factors for *R equi* infection.[5] The role that exhaled *R equi* has in the epidemiology of *R equi* infection remains to be determined.[6] Virulent and avirulent strains of *R equi* exist and both are commonly isolated from horse manure, air, and soil in equine farms.[7] Virulent strains carry a virulence plasmid and express a highly immunogenic surface protein called virulence-associated protein A (VapA). This protein is required for intracellular survival of the bacterium inside macrophages. Strains lacking the *vapA* gene cannot successfully replicate inside the macrophage and therefore are considered avirulent to foals.[8] Most clinically affected foals carry vapA-positive strains but clinical samples should be tested for the presence of the *vapA* gene to confirm virulence.

PATHOGENESIS OF *RHODOCOCCUS EQUI*

R equi does not affect adult horses unless these are immunocompromised. To date, which specific age-related factors are responsible for this susceptibility remains to be determined. Immunosuppressed people, cats, camelids, and dogs are also susceptible to infection.[9–12]

Early on, it was assumed that foals were infected closer to the development of clinical signs (3–6 months of age), time that coincided with the natural decrease of maternal antibodies. The insidious character of the disease along with the ability of foals to compensate for the progressive loss of functional lung,[13] made it hard to identify early age as a risk factor until thoracic ultrasonography made it possible to observe pulmonary lesions as early as 1 month of age in subclinical animals.[14] It is now well established that foals are infected shortly after birth and they become less susceptible as they age.[15–17] Exposure of foals to airborne virulent *R equi* during the first 2 weeks of life is associated with the development of disease[17]; the role oral exposure plays in disease development is unclear. Once inhaled, virulent *R equi* infects alveolar macrophages where the organism replicates until macrophage necrosis occurs. Continuous macrophage death and reinfection of new macrophages leads to the characteristic abscess formation.[13] Similar to *Mycobacterium tuberculosis*, *R equi* is slow growing and clinical signs do not develop for months.[18] This understanding of the time of infection has changed prophylactic and treatment recommendations and has been key for the improvement of research models to study this disease.

Unfortunately, there are no small animal models to replicate this condition. Mice are not susceptible to *R equi* infection unless they are immunocompromised and develop systemic instead of respiratory disease.[19] Guinea pigs seem to be resistant to pulmonary infection with virulent *R equi*.[20] Although some of these nonequine models are useful to perform initial in vitro and in vivo testing,[21] foal models are needed for the final evaluation of prophylactic methods, vaccines, and for the understanding of *R equi* pathogenesis in equids. This situation poses challenges for *R equi* research. Housing of mares and foals is expensive, mare's gestation is long, and foals are not genetically identical, which results in variable results and the need for studies with larger sample sizes.

CLINICAL SIGNS

The clinical signs of *R equi* infection vary with the location of the infection. The pulmonary form, which is the most common presentation, results in clinical signs of pneumonia of variable severity. Early on, foals may develop fever, anorexia, and lethargy, which are followed by tachypnea, increased respiratory effort (nostril flaring), cough, and nasal discharge as the disease progresses.[22] These signs are worse in hot, humid environments.[23] In farms where *R equi* infection is endemic, thoracic ultrasonography reveals rates of subclinical infection (pulmonary lesions consistent with abscessation or consolidation in foals without clinical signs) above 50% of the foal population. Without treatment, 70% to 85% of these foals will remain subclinical and will heal over time.[24] However, 20% to 25% of these foals will develop clinical signs of pneumonia that requires treatment.[7,24,25] Overall, uncomplicated pulmonary infection carries a high survival rate (>90%) but severe pneumonia may result in higher mortality rates (19%).[23]

Extrapulmonary lesions are not uncommon and can affect a wide variety of organ systems. Moreover, multiple systems may be affected at once. Thus, it is important to closely evaluate extrapulmonary sites in foals with suspected or confirmed *R equi* infection. *R equi* bacteremia may be responsible for these presentations but an association between a positive blood culture and a specific extrapulmonary presentation has not been found.[26] Abdominal manifestations, the most common extrapulmonary presentation, can cause severe disease and high mortality rate. Foals usually present with diarrhea, fever, anorexia, and lethargy and may have leukopenia and hypoproteinemia because of granulomatous enterocolitis or enterotyphlocolitis. Milder forms present with soft manure, poor growth rates, and rough haircoat. Abdominal lymphadenitis is typically detected postmortem but may occasionally be visible on abdominal ultrasonography. Abdominal abscessation can lead to septic peritonitis.[26] Subclinical pyogranulomatous hepatitis has also been identified during necropsy.[26] Both, immune-mediated and septic polysynovitis can occur because of *R equi* infection. Foals with immune-mediated polysynovitis have effusion in multiple joints but no signs of lameness and respond well to corticosteroid treatment.[27] In contrast, foals with septic joint/s or osteomyelitis are lame and require aggressive treatment. Unilateral or bilateral uveitis, defined as the presence of aqueous flare, fibrin hypopyon, and/or hyphema, has been described in infected foals and may result from septic or immune-mediated processes.[26–29] Although foals with severe uveitis were less likely to survive, more studies are needed before this clinical finding can be used as a definitive prognosticator.[28] Immune-mediated hemolytic anemia has also been reported.[29,30] Vertebral body osteomyelitis can present with a variety of neurologic signs depending on lesion location. Other presentations such as mediastinal lymphadenopathy, pericarditis, subclinical granulomatous meningitis are less common.[26]

DIAGNOSIS

Early diagnosis of *R equi* is key for successful treatment because this organism responds poorly to routinely used antimicrobials such as beta-lactam and aminoglycoside combinations, or potentiated sulfonamides.[31] Differentiation of *R equi* from other causes of bacterial pneumonia based solely on clinical signs is not possible because the clinical signs are nonspecific to *R equi*. Presumptive diagnosis can be made based on signalment, farm history of *R equi* infection, clinical signs, thoracic ultrasonography, or radiography as well as bloodwork changes.[23] However, a definitive diagnosis can only be achieved by culture and fluid analysis of a tracheobronchial aspirate (TBA) in cases of pneumonia or by culture of a sample obtained from an extrapulmonary site. *R equi* pneumonia can be confirmed if the TBA sample is positive for virulent *R equi* and cytology is consistent with suppurative inflammation. A sterile TBA can be collected percutaneously or using a double-guarded aspiration catheter via endoscopy. Disadvantages of TBA fluid collection are the time required for bacterial culture (72 hours) and the procedural risks in cases of severe respiratory disease.[23] Bronchoalveolar lavage fluid (BALF) collection is easily performed in the field. Cytological evaluation of BALF from foals with *R equi* pneumonia had a higher neutrophil percentage than foals with other causes of bacterial pneumonia. However, the large overlap in the range of neutrophil percentage between both groups limits the diagnostic use of this test.[32]

Imaging of the lungs is useful to detect pulmonary pathologic condition and aids presumptive diagnosis. Thoracic radiographs of foals with *R equi* pneumonia show ill-defined soft tissue nodules with or without irregular areas of cavitation.[33] Superficial pulmonary abscessation and consolidation are also easily identifiable using thoracic ultrasonography.[33] Although these changes are common in foals with clinical and subclinical pneumonia, they are not pathognomonic for *R equi*. Radiographic evidence of thoracic abscessation in pneumonic foals showed a sensitivity of 71% and a specificity of 85% for the diagnosis of *R equi* pneumonia.[23] Bloodwork changes are nonpathognomonic for *R equi* pneumonia either. Leukocytosis characterized by mature neutrophilia and monocytosis, as well as high fibrinogen and globulin concentrations, are common in clinical and subclinical *R equi* infection.[23,34] Thus, bloodwork should not be used in isolation to decide the treatment of foals. These results are best used in combination with other parameters to promote targeted foal treatment.[35,36] Serum amyloid A (SAA) was not a reliable predictor of clinical *R equi* pneumonia in a study with a low number of foals but it was useful to evaluate disease progression and response to treatment.[37]

Other diagnostic tests, such as real-time quantitative polymerase chain reaction (qPCR) detection of virulent (VapA$^+$) *R equi* in feces, are being evaluated.[38] Fecal qPCR is a noninvasive, rapid diagnostic test but the presence of virulent *R equi* in the manure of normal and subclinical foals poses a challenge for its interpretation.[38] Serology should not be used as a screening tool in farms with endemic *R equi* because positive results will lead to unnecessary treatment of foals.[34] Serum IgG(T) was significantly higher in foals that developed *R equi* pneumonia after experimental and natural infection but more work under field conditions is needed before it can be recommended as a useful marker.[39]

Diagnosis of extrapulmonary lesions can be challenging depending on location and clinical signs. Extrapulmonary lesions should be suspected in foals from endemic farms that have bloodwork changes supportive of chronic infection (mature neutrophilia, monocytosis, thrombocytosis as well as increased SSA, fibrinogen, and globulins). Some lesions may only be recognized on postmortem evaluation.[26] Whenever accessible, samples should be collected and submitted for culture.

TREATMENT

Although there is no question that foals with clinical signs of *R equi* infection should be treated, the equine practitioner is faced with the challenge of deciding when to treat foals with subclinical disease (foals with ultrasonographic or bloodwork evidence of infection but without clinical signs of disease). Many farms with endemic *R equi* problems attempt to minimize the occurrence of rhodococcal pneumonia by early identification of infected foals using thoracic ultrasonography coupled with aggressive antibiotic treatment.[14,40] Although this approach was thought to be beneficial in terms of reducing mortality, it is not without risks. The recommended macrolides used to treat *R equi* infections can cause mild, self-limiting diarrhea,[41] and hyperthermia in foals[42,43] as well as occasionally fatal colitis in mares.[44] Evidence indicates that the prevalence of rhodococcal infections on farms may be overestimated using routine ultrasound screening. Thus, the incidence of *R equi* pneumonia on farms that do not routinely use thoracic ultrasonography varies between 5% and 20%, whereas on farms that use ultrasound screening, the number of foals identified with lung lesions ranged from 29% to 64%.[14,40] These results, along with recent studies, suggest that many foals with small pulmonary lesions recover without antimicrobial therapy and that antimicrobial treatment of foals with small lesions (median abscess score ≤6–10 cm) does not significantly accelerate lesion resolution relative to administration of a placebo.[22,24,41]

More farms are now introducing treatment protocol changes with the goal of minimizing the number of foals that receive antimicrobials every year. Alteration of the treatment criteria to exclude foals with subclinical disease and small ultrasonographic lesions decreased the number of foals treated from 80% to 50% without increasing mortality in a farm.[36] In another farm, the addition of white blood cells and SSA to a thoracic ultrasonographic screening program reduced the number of foals treated without significantly increasing the risk of the development of clinical *R equi* pneumonia.[35] Establishing this type of program in a farm that uses a screen and treat program may be difficult for the practitioner due to the perceived risk of increased mortality because of the changes.[35] Moreover, there are no specific recommendations that can be applied to all farms at this time. Therefore, each veterinarian should develop an individualized screening program that gradually aims to minimize the number of foals treated on each farm.

A wide range of antimicrobials is active against *R equi* in vitro but only a few of these are effective in vivo likely due to the intracellular nature of this organism.[45] Thus, an appropriate antimicrobial treatment plan should be used for clinical cases with a presumptive diagnosis of *R equi* pneumonia, because this organism responds poorly to routine antimicrobials, such as beta-lactam and aminoglycoside combinations, or potentiated sulfonamides.[31] Foals 2 to 6 months of age with clinical signs of pneumonia and high white cell count (>20,000 cells/μL) and elevated fibrinogen concentration (>700 mg/dL) are likely to be infected with *R equi* (specificity 85%).[34] Mixed bacterial infections, most commonly with *Streptococcus* spp. and *Actinobacillus* spp., are not uncommon in foals with moderate-to-severe *R equi* pneumonia[23] but co-infection does not seem to negatively influence prognosis.[46] Mixed bacterial infections are rarer in mild-to-moderate *R equi* pneumonia cases.[32,46]

The recommended treatment of *R equi* infection is a combination of a macrolide and rifampin (5 mg/kg PO Q12 h or 10 mg/kg PO q24 h). Clarithromycin (7.5 mg/kg PO Q12 h) and azithromycin (10 mg/kg PO Q24 h for 5 days, Q48 h thereafter) are the most commonly used macrolides. Although administration of rifampin decreases oral absorption and plasma concentration of clarithromycin in foals,[47] the concentration of these drugs in pulmonary epithelial lining fluid and in pulmonary macrophages of foals remains above the minimum inhibitory concentration for *R equi* when this combination is used.[48,49] Moreover, the combination of drugs was found to be superior than monotherapy in mice.[50] Typically, antimicrobials are administered for 4 to 8 weeks[51] but duration of treatment varies with disease presentation and shorter courses may be beneficial.[52] Because the combination treatment can be expensive and labor intensive, drugs that can be used for monotherapy have been investigated. Tulathromycin, a macrolide that is given intramuscularly once a week (2.5 mg/kg) does not seem to be effective when used alone[25,53] but was shown to have similar treatment efficacy as the azithromycin–rifampin combination in foals with mild to moderate to severe pneumonia when combined with oral rifampin (10 mg/kg Q24 h).[52] Intramuscular administration of gamithromycin (6 mg/kg, IM, once a week) was shown to be noninferior to azithromycin–rifampin. However, almost 60% of the foals developed significant side effects including colic that required treatment with analgesics and marked lameness. Local pain that lasted for 5 days was also observed when the drug was administered subcutaneously.[54,55] Intravenous gamithromycin (6 mg/kg, IV, once a week) through a catheter induces significantly fewer adverse effects but more research in needed to refine the dose and dosing interval in foals with R equi.[49,55] Additional research is needed before monotherapy can be recommended in moderate-to-severe R equi cases.

Aside from the described side effects related to local site of administration, macrolides cause diarrhea in a third of the treated foals. Although the diarrhea usually improves with treatment discontinuation, a subset of these foals may require supportive treatment; therefore, diarrheic foals should be closely monitored.[56] Foals should be kept in well-ventilated, cold areas while treated with macrolides. Macrolides cause a drug-induced anhidrosis, which in turn results in hyperthermia that may be fatal. Hyperthermic foals are usually tachypneic. Anhidrosis develops shortly after treatment is initiated and lasts for at least 3 weeks after discontinuation of treatment.[42,43] Increased liver enzymes may be observed in foals that receive rifampin.[24] An in-depth review of R equi treatment has been published recently.[51]

The efficacy of other drugs for the treatment of R equi has been investigated. When used as monotherapy, doxycycline failed to reduce the size of lung abscesses compared to other drugs and to placebo groups in experimental animal studies.[22] The combination of doxycycline and azithromycin had a similar therapeutic effect compared with the combination of rifampin and azithromycin in a randomized controlled clinical trial in foals with mild or subclinical pneumonia.[41] The study did not include an azithromycin group; thus, it is difficult to assess the real contribution of doxycycline to the combination. Gentamicin was shown to be among the most active drugs against R equi using an in vitro intracellular bactericidal assay[45] but failed to reach the mutant prevention concentrations in BAL cells and pulmonary fluid lining.[57] Intravenous liposomal gentamicin was effective for the treatment of R equi pneumonia after experimental infection but caused nephrotoxicity in 50% of the treated foals.[58] Alternative routes such as nebulization or different dosing intervals will be needed before this drug can be safely used in these foals.[58] The use of gallium maltolate is not recommended for treatment at this time because its efficacy in clinical cases has not been demonstrated.[59]

IMPACT OF SCREENING ON *RHODOCOCCUS EQUI* RESISTANCE

Prophylactic antimicrobial treatment of foals with subclinical lesions is not superior to the use of a placebo[22] and has led to a significant increase in AMR strains.[60–62] Farms that prophylactically treated foals based on thoracic ultrasonography screening programs had significantly higher concentrations of AMR strains in their soil than farms that did not routinely treat subclinical foals.[63] Resistance has also significantly increased in clinical samples from foals. Reports of resistance ranged from 0.7% to 3.7% before 2010 in studies from KY and Texas.[64,65] This number increased to 13% resistance for rifampin and 16% resistance to macrolides between 2007 and 2017 in KY.[65] Virulent R equi isolates resistant to rifampicin and macrolides were more common in necropsied foals previously treated with mainstay dual therapy than in foals that did not receive any antimicrobial treatment.[66]

The development of AMR strains has multiple clinical implications. Macrolide resistance in macrolide-resistant isolates of *R equi* in the United States is caused by erm(46), an erythromycin-resistant methylase gene that has been identified only in *R equi* to date.[67,68] Strains that express the gene for resistance are resistant to all macrolides, lincosamides, and streptogramin B,[65] and the gene could transfer horizontally to other bacterium.[69] Foals that harbor resistant strains contaminate the environment via cough or manure. Treatment options are greatly minimized in phase of resistance. Alternative antimicrobials to treat AMR *R equi* infections such as imipenem are limited by their use in human medicine.[70] Moreover, this drug does not seem to achieve therapeutic concentrations in BAL cells or pulmonary lining fluid.[57] The limitations of other antimicrobials have been described in the treatment section. Survival of foals infected with resistant strains is significantly lower than survival of foals infected with antimicrobial susceptible strains.[65] When treated with a rifampin-macrolide combination, only 25% of the foals infected with a resistant strain survived to discharge in comparison with 69% survival rate for the foals infected with a nonresistant strain.[65] Epidemiological studies are needed to determine the duration of AMR persistence on farms and the possibility of resistance sharing between bacteria that might serve as a repository of antimicrobial-resistance genes that could threaten public health.[63]

PREVENTION

It is important to understand that absolute prevention of *R equi* infection is unlikely. Thus, even with a successful prophylactic program in place, foals are likely to develop pulmonary lesions identifiable using thoracic ultrasonography. The goal of a prophylactic program should be to decrease the incidence of clinical pneumonia and its severity because this will minimize the use of antimicrobials and the development of AMR strains.

To date, there is no commercially available vaccine to prevent infection against *R equi* or to minimize the frequency of clinical disease. Vaccination of neonatal foals is challenging because priming of the naïve neonatal immune system requires multiple vaccine doses.[71] As foals are infected shortly after birth,[7,16] complete vaccination will only be achieved after infection has occurred. Moreover, vaccine response may be affected by the presence of maternal antibodies.[72] Multiple vaccine candidates have been tested and failed to prevent infection in foals or have been only tested in nonequine models. A detailed summary of this early vaccine study has been published elsewhere.[72] A recent study evaluating a pilus (Rpl) vaccine administered during gestation to mares failed to decrease the severity of pneumonia in foals after experimental infection in spite of higher colostral antibodies against the pilus in vaccinated mares and higher serum and BALF antibody titers in foals born from vaccinated mares.[73] A vaccine based on a highly conserved bacterial polysaccharide (poly-N-acetylglucosamine or PNAG) was protective against intrabronchial challenge of 28-day-old foals[71] but failed to reduce the incidence of pneumonia in foals challenged shortly after birth.[74] As of now, the only vaccination method that protected foals against *R equi* after experimental infection was the administration of live, virulent *R equi* orally.[75] However, electron beam-inactivated *R equi*, which are structurally intact microorganisms, did not reduce the proportion of foals developing clinical pneumonia after experimental challenge.[76]

Because of the current vaccine situation, most farms with endemic *R equi* rely on *R equi*-specific hyperimmune plasma (Re-HIP) administration as a means for prophylaxis. Early research reported mixed results with this practice[77–80] but newer data support its use based on clinical benefits. Intravenous administration of Re-Hip to neonates significantly reduced the severity of pneumonia after experimental challenge of 1-week-old foals.[81] Administration of a novel hyperimmune plasma, raised against β-1→6-poly-N-acetyl glucosamine (PNAG-HIP) shortly after birth was not superior to a commercially available Re-HIP product for protecting foals against natural development of R equi pneumonia.[82] Recently, the volume of Re-HIP administered has been evaluated. Foals that received 2 L of Re-HIP shortly after birth were 2.4 times less likely to develop clinical pneumonia than foals that received 1 L of Re-HIP at the same time. Transfusion of 2 L of Re-HIP also resulted in a lower proportion of foals (12% vs 32%) developing subclinical pneumonia identified by thoracic ultrasonography.[83] Moreover, the administration of 2 L of Re-HIP appeared safe.[83,84] More research evaluating the effect of the volume and time of Re-HIP administration is needed as the 2 studies previously described are limited by their retrospective nature. Foals that received Re-HIP shed less-virulent R equi in their manure when compared with foals that did not receive Re-HIP after experimental infection.[85] Additional research is needed to assess the potential benefit of Re-HIP administration in environmental contamination. Another area that requires further investigation is the mechanism of Re-HIP protection. It is tempting to speculate that R equi-specific antibodies are fully responsible for the acquired protection because the amount and activity of antibodies in Re-HIP are positively associated with the protection against R equi[86]; however, the role other proteins, such as complement, has been shown to be key for R equi opsonization.[71] Although recommended at this time, hyperimmune plasma administration is expensive, labor intensive, and mild side effects such as tachycardia, tachypnea, or hyperthermia, which may require the transfusion to be slowed down or discontinued, may occur.[87] Moreover, there is a large variation in the amount of antibodies present in Re-HIP between companies and among bags of the same lot number, which leads to variable amount of antibody levels after plasma administration.[88]

In summary, R equi infection is a common condition of foals typically characterized by self-resolving subclinical pneumonia. A subset (20%–30%) of infected foals will develop more severe disease and will require treatment. Extrapulmonary infection has a variable prognosis depending on the location of the infection. The challenge in the years to come is to develop better biomarkers of disease that may result in strategic antimicrobial use. Targeted treatment is imperative in face of the growing antimicrobial resistance seen in R equi. Prevention strategies such as the development of protective vaccines and the improvement of products used for passive immunization are also needed. Research in these areas is challenging because of our incomplete understanding of this disease and the need for foal-based research.

CLINICS CARE POINTS

- Pulmonary lesions seen on ultrasound without other clinical signs does not warrant antimicrobial treatment.
- Treat R. equi with a macrolide - rifampin combination unless resistance is documented.
- Intravenous administration of plasma shortly after birth appears to decrease disease severity.
- There is no information about which foals will develop clinical disease.

REFERENCES

1. Muscatello G. Rhodococcus equi pneumonia in the foal–part 1: pathogenesis and epidemiology. Vet J 2012;192(1):20–6.
2. Cohen ND. Causes of and farm management factors associated with disease and death in foals. J Am Vet Med Assoc 1994;204(10):1644–51.
3. Barton MD, Hughes KL. Ecology of Rhodococcus equi. Vet Microbiol 1984;9(1): 65–76.
4. Pusterla N, Wilson WD, Mapes S, et al. Diagnostic evaluation of real-time PCR in the detection of Rhodococcus equi in faeces and nasopharyngeal swabs from foals with pneumonia. Vet Rec 2007;161(8):272–5.
5. Chaffin MK, Cohen ND, Martens RJ. Evaluation of equine breeding farm characteristics as risk factors for development of Rhodococcus equi pneumonia in foals. J Am Vet Med Assoc 2003;222(4):467–75.
6. Muscatello G, Gilkerson JR, Browning GF. Detection of virulent Rhodococcus equi in exhaled air samples from naturally infected foals. J Clin Microbiol 2009; 47(3):734–7.
7. Cohen ND, Chaffin MK, Kuskie KR, et al. Association of perinatal exposure to airborne Rhodococcus equi with risk of pneumonia caused by R equi in foals. Am J Vet Res 2013;74(1):102–9.
8. Jain S, Bloom BR, Hondalus MK. Deletion of vapA encoding Virulence Associated Protein A attenuates the intracellular actinomycete Rhodococcus equi. Mol Microbiol 2003;50(1):115–28.
9. Aslam MW, Lau SF, Chin CSL, et al. Clinicopathological and radiographic features in 40 cats diagnosed with pulmonary and cutaneous Rhodococcus equi infection (2012-2018). J Feline Med Surg 2020;22(8):774–90.
10. Lin WV, Kruse RL, Yang K, et al. Diagnosis and management of pulmonary infection due to Rhodococcus equi. Clin Microbiol Infect 2019;25(3):310–5.
11. Bryan LK, Clark SD, Diaz-Delgado J, et al. Rhodococcus equi Infections in Dogs. Vet Pathol 2017;54(1):159–63.
12. Kinne J, Madarame H, Takai S, et al. Disseminated Rhodococcus equi infection in dromedary camels (Camelus dromedarius). Vet Microbiol 2011;149(1–2):269–72.
13. Vazquez-Boland JA, Giguere S, Hapeshi A, et al. Rhodococcus equi: the many facets of a pathogenic actinomycete. Vet Microbiol 2013;167(1–2):9–33.
14. Slovis NM, McCracken JL, Mundy G. How to use thoracic ultrasound to screen foals for Rhodococcus equi at affected farms. . Paper presented at: American Association of Equine Practitioners Annual Conference2005; Lexington, KY
15. Horowitz ML, Cohen ND, Takai S, et al. Application of Sartwell's model (lognormal distribution of incubation periods) to age at onset and age at death of foals with Rhodococcus equi pneumonia as evidence of perinatal infection. J Vet Intern Med 2001;15(3):171–5.
16. Sanz M, Loynachan A, Sun L, et al. The effect of bacterial dose and foal age at challenge on Rhodococcus equi infection. Vet Microbiol 2013;167(3–4):623–31.
17. Cohen ND, Kuskie KR, Smith JL, et al. Association of airborne concentration of virulent Rhodococcus equi with location (stall versus paddock) and month (January through June) on 30 horse breeding farms in central Kentucky. Am J Vet Res 2012;73(10):1603–9.
18. Hondalus MK. Pathogenesis and virulence of Rhodococcus equi. Vet Microbiol 1997;56(3–4):257–68.

19. Phumoonna T, Barton MD, Vanniasinkam T, et al. Chimeric vapA/groEL2 DNA vaccines enhance clearance of Rhodococcus equi in aerosol challenged C3H/He mice. Vaccine 2008;26(20):2457–65.

20. Bordin AI, Gressler LT, Alexander ERC, et al. Guinea pig infection with the intracellular pathogen Rhodococcus equi. Vet Microbiol 2018;215:18–22.

21. Gonzalez-Iglesias P, Scortti M, MacArthur I, et al. Mouse lung infection model to assess Rhodococcus equi virulence and vaccine protection. Vet Microbiol 2014; 172(1–2):256–64.

22. Venner M, Rodiger A, Laemmer M, et al. Failure of antimicrobial therapy to accelerate spontaneous healing of subclinical pulmonary abscesses on a farm with endemic infections caused by Rhodococcus equi. Vet J 2012;192(3):293–8.

23. Leclere M, Magdesian KG, Kass PH, et al. Comparison of the clinical, microbiological, radiological and haematological features of foals with pneumonia caused by Rhodococcus equi and other bacteria. Vet J 2011;187(1):109–12.

24. Venner M, Astheimer K, Lammer M, et al. Efficacy of mass antimicrobial treatment of foals with subclinical pulmonary abscesses associated with Rhodococcus equi. J Vet Intern Med 2013;27(1):171–6.

25. Venner M, Credner N, Lammer M, et al. Comparison of tulathromycin, azithromycin and azithromycin-rifampin for the treatment of mild pneumonia associated with Rhodococcus equi. Vet Rec 2013;173(16):397.

26. Reuss SM, Chaffin MK, Cohen ND. Extrapulmonary disorders associated with Rhodococcus equi infection in foals: 150 cases (1987-2007). J Am Vet Med Assoc 2009;235(7):855–63.

27. Huber L, Giguere S, Berghaus LJ, et al. Development of septic polysynovitis and uveitis in foals experimentally infected with Rhodococcus equi. PLoS One 2018; 13(2):e0192655.

28. Tarancon I, Leiva M, Jose-Cunilleras E, et al. Ophthalmologic findings associated with Rhodococcus equi bronchopneumonia in foals. Vet Ophthalmol 2019;22(5): 660–5.

29. Wilkes EJA, Hughes KL, Kessell AE, et al. Successful management of multiple extrapulmonary complications associated with Rhodococcus equi pneumonia in a foal. Equine Vet Education 2016;4:186–92.

30. Johns IC, Desrochers A, Wotman KL, et al. Presumed immune-mediated hemolytic anemia in two foals with Rhodococcus equi infection. J Vet Emerg Crit Care (San Antonio) 2011;21(3):273–8.

31. Sweeney CR, Sweeney RW, Divers TJ. Rhodococcus-Equi Pneumonia in 48 Foals - Response to Antimicrobial Therapy. Vet Microbiol 1987;14(3):329–36.

32. Vitale V, Sgorbini M, Cuteri V, et al. Cytological Findings in Bronchoalveolar Lavage Fluid of Foals With Pneumonia Caused by Rhodococcus equi and Other Bacteria. J Equine Vet Sci 2019;79:9–12.

33. Ramirez S, Lester GD, Roberts GR. Diagnostic contribution of thoracic ultrasonography in 17 foals with Rhodococcus equi pneumonia. Vet Radiol Ultrasound 2004;45(2):172–6.

34. Giguere S, Hernandez J, Gaskin J, et al. Evaluation of white blood cell concentration, plasma fibrinogen concentration, and an agar gel immunodiffusion test for early identification of foals with Rhodococcus equi pneumonia. J Am Vet Med Assoc 2003;222(6):775–81.

35. McCracken JL. Evaluation of white blood cell, fibrinogen, serum amyloid A adn ultrasonographic grade to refine a R. equi screening program. Paper presented at: 65th American Association of Equine Practitioners Annual Convention2019; Denver, CO.

36. Arnold-Lehna D, Venner M, Berghaus LJ, et al. Changing policy to treat foals with Rhodococcus equi pneumonia in the later course of disease decreases antimicrobial usage without increasing mortality rate. Equine Vet J 2020;52(4):531–7.
37. Passamonti F, Vardi DM, Stefanetti V, et al. Rhodococcus equi pneumonia in foals: an assessment of the early diagnostic value of serum amyloid A and plasma fibrinogen concentrations in equine clinical practice. Vet J 2015;203(2):211–8.
38. Shaw SD, Cohen ND, Chaffin MK, et al. Estimating the Sensitivity and Specificity of Real-Time Quantitative PCR of Fecal Samples for Diagnosis of Rhodococcus equi Pneumonia in Foals. J Vet Intern Med 2015;29(6):1712–7.
39. Sanz MG, Villarino N, Ferreira-Oliveira A, et al. VapA-specific IgG and IgG subclasses responses after natural infection and experimental challenge of foals with Rhodococcus equi. Vet Immunol Immunopathol 2015;164(1–2):10–5.
40. McCranken JL, Slovis NM. Use of thoracic ultrasound for the prevention of Rhodococcus equi pneumonia on endemic farms. Paper presented at: American Association of Equine Practitioners Annual Conference2009; Las Vegas, Nevada.
41. Wetzig M, Venner M, Giguere S. Efficacy of the combination of doxycycline and azithromycin for the treatment of foals with mild to moderate bronchopneumonia. Equine Vet J 2020;52(4):613–9.
42. Stieler AL, Sanchez LC, Mallicote MF, et al. Macrolide-induced hyperthermia in foals: Role of impaired sweat responses. Equine Vet J 2016;48(5):590–4.
43. Stieler Stewart AL, Sanchez LC, Mallicote MF, et al. Effects of clarithromycin, azithromycin and rifampicin on terbutaline-induced sweating in foals. Equine Vet J 2017;49(5):624–8.
44. Baverud V, Franklin A, Gunnarsson A, et al. Clostridium difficile associated with acute colitis in mares when their foals are treated with erythromycin and rifampicin for Rhodococcus equi pneumonia. Equine Vet J 1998;30(6):482–8.
45. Giguere S, Berghaus LJ, Lee EA. Activity of 10 antimicrobial agents against intracellular Rhodococcus equi. Vet Microbiol 2015;178(3–4):275–8.
46. Giguere S, Jordan LM, Glass K, et al. Relationship of mixed bacterial infection to prognosis in foals with pneumonia caused by Rhodococcus equi. J Vet Intern Med 2012;26(6):1443–8.
47. Peters J, Block W, Oswald S, et al. Oral absorption of clarithromycin is nearly abolished by chronic comedication of rifampicin in foals. Drug Metab Dispos 2011;39(9):1643–9.
48. Berlin S, Kirschbaum A, Spieckermann L, et al. Pharmacological indices and pulmonary distribution of rifampicin after repeated oral administration in healthy foals. Equine Vet J 2017;49(5):618–23.
49. Berlin S, Spieckermann L, Oswald S, et al. Pharmacokinetics and Pulmonary Distribution of Clarithromycin and Rifampicin after Concomitant and Consecutive Administration in Foals. Mol Pharmacol 2016;13(3):1089–99.
50. Burton AJ, Giguere S, Berghaus LJ, et al. Activity of clarithromycin or rifampin alone or in combination against experimental Rhodococcus equi infection in mice. Antimicrobial Agents Chemother 2015;59(6):3633–6.
51. Giguere S. Treatment of Infections Caused by Rhodococcus equi. Vet Clin North Am Equine Pract 2017;33(1):67–85.
52. Goebel B, Freise F, Venner M. Comparison of the efficacy of rifampin/azithromycin and rifampin/tulathromycin for the treatment of foals affected with pneumonia. Equine Vet Education 2022;34:e73–7.
53. Rutenberg D, Venner M, Giguere S. Efficacy of Tulathromycin for the Treatment of Foals with Mild to Moderate Bronchopneumonia. J Vet Intern Med 2017;31(3):901–6.

54. Hildebrand F, Venner M, Giguere S. Efficacy of gamithromycin for the treatment of foals with mild to moderate bronchopneumonia. J Vet Intern Med 2015;29(1): 333–8.

55. Hildebrand F, Giguere S, Venner M. Treatment with gamithromycin in foals with pneumonia: comparative efficacy and adverse effects of i.m. versus i.v. administration. Pferdeheilkunde 2015;31:165–70.

56. Giguere S, Jacks S, Roberts GD. Retrospective comparison of azithromycin, clarithromycin, and erythromycin for the treatment of foals with Rhodococcus equi pneumonia. J Vet Intern Med 2004;18:568–73.

57. Berghaus LJ, Giguere S, Guldbech K. Mutant prevention concentration and mutant selection window for 10 antimicrobial agents against Rhodococcus equi. Vet Microbiol 2013;166(3–4):670–5.

58. Cohen ND, Giguere S, Burton AJ, et al. Use of Liposomal Gentamicin for Treatment of 5 Foals with Experimentally Induced Rhodococcus equi Pneumonia. J Vet Intern Med 2016;30(1):322–5.

59. Giguere S, Cohen N. Controversies in therapy of infections caused by Rhodococcus equi in foals. Equine Vet Education 2018;30(6):336–41.

60. Burton AJ, Giguere S, Sturgill TL, et al. Macrolide- and rifampin-resistant Rhodococcus equi on a horse breeding farm, Kentucky, USA. Emerg Infect Dis 2013; 19(2):282–5.

61. Huber L, Giguere S, Cohen ND, et al. Prevalence and risk factors associated with emergence of Rhodococcus equi resistance to macrolides and rifampicin in horse-breeding farms in Kentucky, USA. Vet Microbiol 2019;235:243–7.

62. Alvarez-Narvaez S, Giguere S, Cohen N, et al. Spread of Multidrug-Resistant Rhodococcus equi, United States. Emerg Infect Dis 2021;27(2):529–37.

63. Huber L, Giguere S, Hart KA, et al. Association between antimicrobial treatment of subclinical pneumonia in foals and selection of macrolide- and rifampicin-resistant Rhodococcus equi strains at horse-breeding farms in central Kentucky. J Am Vet Med Assoc 2021;258(6):648–53.

64. Giguere S, Lee E, Williams E, et al. Determination of the prevalence of antimicrobial resistance to macrolide antimicrobials or rifampin in Rhodococcus equi isolates and treatment outcome in foals infected with antimicrobial-resistant isolates of R equi. J Am Vet Med Assoc 2010;237(1):74–81.

65. Huber L, Giguere S, Slovis NM, et al. Emergence of Resistance to Macrolides and Rifampin in Clinical Isolates of Rhodococcus equi from Foals in Central Kentucky, 1995 to 2017. Antimicrobial Agents Chemother 2019;63(1). e01714–18.

66. Erol E, Locke S, Saied A, et al. Antimicrobial susceptibility patterns of Rhodococcus equi from necropsied foals with rhodococcosis. Vet Microbiol 2020;242: 108568.

67. Asoh N, Watanabe H, Fines-Guyon M, et al. Emergence of rifampin-resistant Rhodococcus equi with several types of mutations in the rpoB gene among AIDS patients in northern Thailand. J Clin Microbiol 2003;41(6):2337–40.

68. Giguere S, Berghaus LJ, Willingham-Lane JM. Antimicrobial Resistance in Rhodococcus equi. Microbiol Spectr 2017;5(5). ARBA 0004-22016.

69. Alvarez-Narvaez S, Giguere S, Berghaus LJ, et al. Horizontal Spread of Rhodococcus equi Macrolide Resistance Plasmid pRErm46 across Environmental Actinobacteria. Appl Environ Microbiol 2020;86(9). e00108-20.

70. Gundelly P, Suzuki Y, Ribes JA, et al. Differences in Rhodococcus equi Infections Based on Immune Status and Antibiotic Susceptibility of Clinical Isolates in a Case Series of 12 Patients and Cases in the Literature. Biomed Res Int 2016; 2016:2737295.

71. Cywes-Bentley C, Rocha JN, Bordin AI, et al. Antibody to Poly-N-acetyl glucosamine provides protection against intracellular pathogens: Mechanism of action and validation in horse foals challenged with Rhodococcus equi. PLoS Pathog 2018;14(7):e1007160.

72. Giles C, Vanniasinkam T, Ndi S, et al. Rhodococcus equi (Prescottella equi) vaccines; the future of vaccine development. Equine Vet J 2015;47(5):510–8.

73. Cesar FB. Rhodococcus equi in the foal –improving diagnostic and prevention measures - theses and dissertations: veterinary sciences 2018. Available at. https://uknowledge.uky.edu/gluck_etds/36UniversityofKentucky.

74. Cohen ND, Kahn SK, Cywes-Bentley C, et al. Serum Antibody Activity against Poly-N-Acetyl Glucosamine (PNAG), but Not PNAG Vaccination Status, Is Associated with Protecting Newborn Foals against Intrabronchial Infection with Rhodococcus equi. Microbiol Spectr 2021;9(1):e0063821.

75. Hooper-McGrevy KE, Wilkie BN, Prescott JF. Virulence-associated protein-specific serum immunoglobulin G-isotype expression in young foals protected against Rhodococcus equi pneumonia by oral immunization with virulent R. Equi Vaccin 2005;23(50):5760–7.

76. Rocha JN, Cohen ND, Bordin AI, et al. Oral Administration of Electron-Beam Inactivated Rhodococcus equi Failed to Protect Foals against Intrabronchial Infection with Live, Virulent R. equi. PLoS One. 2016;11(2):e0148111.

77. Becu T, Polledo G, Gaskin JM. Immunoprophylaxis of Rhodococcus equi pneumonia in foals. Vet Microbiol 1997;56(3–4):193–204.

78. Caston SS, McClure SR, Martens RJ, et al. Effect of hyperimmune plasma on the severity of pneumonia caused by Rhodococcus equi in experimentally infected foals. Vet Ther 2006;7(4):361–75.

79. Madigan JE, Hietala S, Muller N. Protection against naturally acquired Rhodococcus equi pneumonia in foals by administration of hyperimmune plasma. J Reprod Fertil Suppl 1991;44:571–8.

80. Perkins GA, Yeager A, Erb HN, et al. Survival of foals with experimentally induced Rhodococcus equi infection given either hyperimmune plasma containing R. equi antibody or normal equine plasma. Vet Ther 2002;3(3):334–46.

81. Sanz MG, Loynachan A, Horohov DW. Rhodococcus equi hyperimmune plasma decreases pneumonia severity after a randomised experimental challenge of neonatal foals. Vet Rec 2016;178(11):261.

82. Kahn SK, Cywes-Bentley C, Blodgett GP, et al. Randomized, controlled trial comparing Rhodococcus equi and poly-N-acetyl glucosamine hyperimmune plasma to prevent R equi pneumonia in foals. J Vet Intern Med 2021;35(6):2912–9.

83. Kahn SK, Blodgett GP, Canaday NM, et al. Transfusion With 2 L of Hyperimmune Plasma is Superior to Transfusion of 1 L or Less for Protecting Foals Against Subclinical Pneumonia Attributed to Rhodococcus equi. J Equine Vet Sci 2019;79:54–8.

84. Flores-Ahlschwede P, Kahn SK, Ahlschwede S, et al. Transfusion with 2 litres of hyperimmune plasma is superior to transfusion of 1 litre for protecting foals against pneumonia attributed to Rhodococcus equi. Equine Vet J 2021;34(1):e67–72.

85. Sanz MG, Bradway DS, Horohov DW, et al. Rhodococcus equi-specific hyperimmune plasma administration decreases faecal shedding of pathogenic R. equi in foals. Vet Rec 2019;185(1):19.

86. Kahn SK, Cywes-Bentley C, Blodgett GP, et al. Antibody activities in hyperimmune plasma against the Rhodococcus equi virulence -associated protein A or

poly-N-acetyl glucosamine are associated with protection of foals against rhodo-coccal pneumonia. PLoS One 2021;16(8):e0250133.

87. Hardefeldt LY, Keuler N, Peek SF. Incidence of transfusion reactions to commercial equine plasma. J Vet Emerg Crit Care (San Antonio) 2010;20(4):421–5.

88. Sanz MG, Oliveira AF, Page A, et al. Administration of commercial Rhodococcus equi specific hyperimmune plasma results in variable amounts of IgG against pathogenic bacteria in foals. Vet Rec 2014;175(19):485.

An Overview of Equine Enteric Clostridial Diseases

Deepa Ashwarya Kuttappan, BVSc, AH, MVSc, PhD, DABT[a],
Shankumar Mooyottu, MVSc, BVSc, MS, PhD[b], Brett A. Sponseller, DVM, PhD[c,d],*

KEYWORDS

- Enterocolitis • Clostridial diseases • GI tract • Equine

KEY POINTS

- Adults on antibiotics and neonatal foals appear to have a microbiome favoring growth and establishment of Clostridioides difficile infection.
- Clostridioides difficile causes a pseudomembranous colitis via toxin-mediated mucosal damage of the equine large bowel by production of toxins A and B (TcdA and TcdB) and binary toxin.
- Paeniclostridium sordellii (previously Clostridium sordellii) can cause pseudomembranous enteric disease of the small and large intestine which is mediated largely by lethal toxin (TcsL) and hemorrhagic toxin (TcsH).
- Clostridium perfringens is a genetically heterogeneous anaerobe with a vast array of potential toxins with expression of toxin playing a key role in pathogenicity. C. perfringens type C is commonly reported in foals.
- Tyzzer's disease, a clostridial hepatitis, occurs in foals approximately 6 weeks of age, and is caused by Clostridium piliforme.

INTRODUCTION

Gastrointestinal inflammatory diseases remain an important cause of morbidity and mortality in horses despite many recent advances in monitoring and therapy. Several bacterial and viral causes of enteritis and colitis in adult horses and foals are identified. Enterocolitis associated with the infection due to the genus Clostridia is being discussed here. Clostridia represent a group of rod-shaped, gram-positive, spore-forming anaerobic bacteria that are either soil bacteria or nonpathogenic commensals of the equine GI tract. These commensals form an important component of the healthy

[a] Laboratory Corporation of America, Indianapolis, IN 46250, USA; [b] Department of Pathobiology, Auburn University, College of Veterinary Medicine, 1130 Wire Road, Auburn, AL 36849, USA; [c] Department of Veterinary Microbiology and Preventive Medicine, Iowa State University, 2134 College of Veterinary Medicine, Ames, IA 50011-1134, USA; [d] Department of Veterinary Clinical Sciences, Iowa State University, Ames, IA 50014, USA
* Corresponding author.
E-mail address: baspon@iastate.edu

Vet Clin Equine 39 (2023) 15–23
https://doi.org/10.1016/j.cveq.2022.11.012
0749-0739/23/Crown Copyright © 2022 Published by Elsevier Inc. All rights reserved.
vetequine.theclinics.com

intestinal microflora. Unbalanced dysbiotic conditions of the gut arise due to several factors namely, sudden dietary changes, administration of antimicrobials, stress, procedures such as deworming horses having a heavy parasite load, surgery, or gastric acid suppression. The clostridia responsible for disease will infect the host, overcome the host's immune defenses, grow, multiply in tissues and elaborate their toxins. This has a significant impact on both the well-being of the animal and, adverse economic impact in the case of performance and production animals.

PATHOGENESIS
Clostridioides difficile

Clostridioides difficile is a spore-forming, gram-positive, obligate anaerobe and is capable of surviving in the environment for extended periods of time by way of the spores. The ingested spores sporulate in the digestive tract into the vegetative form of the pathogen, which actively grows and causes infection in the intestinal tract. Owing to the production of toxins, C difficile causes diarrhea and enterocolitis in horses. Both foals and adult horses are equally susceptible to the infection. The highly resistant spore of C difficile is the infectious unit of transmission, which primarily gains entry into the body through the fecal-oral route. The main sources of infection are feces from infected animals, contaminated soil, animal hospitals, and feces of other animals.[1] The organism was first isolated from the meconium of infants and later identified to be a human pathogen[2] and subsequently a pathogen causing enteric disease in humans and animals.

The infectious form of C difficile is the spore, which is highly tolerant of oxygen, disinfectants, and a variety of other stressors and can persist outside of the body for years. In addition, the organism also exists in the stage of vegetative cells. The vegetative form is the active growing state that causes disease in the intestinal tract. It is highly susceptible to oxygen and dies quickly outside the body. The epidemiology and pathophysiology of C difficile infection (CDI) in horses are incompletely understood.

Although a causative agent for colitis, C difficile can also be found in the gut of healthy animals. It is postulated that several factors can increase the risk of disease development by C difficile exposure. Factors that can disrupt the protective normal microflora of the gastrointestinal tract or immunosuppressive agents are associated with the development of CDI. Most authors agree that the two major risk factors for the development of Clostridioides difficile associated disease (CDAD) are antibiotic treatment and hospitalization.[3,4] Yet, in humans, there is increasing recognition of CDI in the absence of any known risk factors.[5,6] Development of CDI involves the proliferation of C difficile in the intestinal tract and the production of C difficile toxins. The primary virulence factors of C difficile are the two major toxins, toxin A (TcdA) and toxin B (TcdB).[7] TcdA has a molecular weight of 308 kDa and toxin B is 269 kDa, and the C-terminal portion of TcdA and TcdB mediates toxin binding to enterocytes.[8] Toxins gain access to the cytoplasm and their enzymatic portions, which have monoglucosyltransferase activity and catalyze glucosylation, inactivating small regulatory proteins of the actin cytoskeleton. This causes disorganization of the cytoskeleton and cell death. The specific function of the toxins is yet to be identified.[9] Some strains of C difficile may also produce an ADP ribosylating binary toxin (CDT) that is made up of two components; CDTa is an enzymatic component and CDTb mediates entry of CDTa into target cells. CDTa ADP-ribosylates G-actin in target cells, disrupting the F-actin:G actin equilibrium and leading to cell death.[9] In CDI, the toxigenicity of the strain determines the severity of infection and thereby the virulence of the strain.[10]

Clostridium perfringens

Clostridium perfringens is found in the environment and the intestinal contents and feces of most humans and animals. The organism is a gram-positive, anaerobic, sporulating rod and is recognized to be the cause of enteric disease in horses of all ages.[11] Horses of all ages are reported to have enteric diseases due to the organism, which are generally noncontagious infections. As the organism is found in the gastrointestinal tract of healthy animals, the predisposing causes to enteric infection by the pathogen are not very well characterized.[12] Being well adapted to the intestinal microenvironment of equids, any disruption to the normal microbiota can lead to overgrowth and infection by the pathogen causing enteritis, enterocolitis, and colitis, manifested clinically by diarrhea and colic of toxigenic origin.[13] Diseases produced by *C perfringens* are mediated by a vast group of toxins, six of which are alpha (CPA), beta (CPB), epsilon (ETX), and iota (ITX), enterotoxin (CPE), and necrotic enteritis like B toxin (NetB). In addition, the toxins that are expressed are used to classify *C perfringens* into seven toxinotypes.[11] Although *C perfringens* types A, B, and C have been associated with enterocolitis in foals, type C is the most commonly reported clostridial enteric pathogen in foals in North America.[14–16] *Clostridium perfringens* type C produces major toxins CPA and CPB. The former is a lecithinase (phospholipase C), which is considered the main virulence factor in *C perfringens* type A-associated myonecrosis in humans and animals. Though type A is associated with enteric infection in horses, the contributing factors are not clearly defined. There are limited reports of disease caused by type B with mostly CPB and ETX toxins.[17–19] Infection can occur by ingesting the spores from a contaminated environment or from infected feces or from the teats of the dam, in the case of foals. The intestinal mucosa is colonized by the bacterium and production and secretion of toxins follows. CPB binds to endothelial cells causing vascular damage, thrombosis, and necrosis directly and induces cell death through the creation of pores in the host cell membrane resulting in an efflux of $K+$ and influx of $Na+$, $Cl-$, and $Ca2+$. Entry of toxins into the systemic circulation is thought to result in death of affected animals.[13,20] Certain type A strains produce NetF toxin that is a β-pore-forming necrotizing toxin belonging to the leukocidin-hemolysin family of toxins, more prevalent in the intestine of horses with enterocolitis than in healthy individuals.[21–23]

Clostridium piliforme

In young foals, Tyzzer's disease (TD) is produced by *Clostridium piliforme*. The organism is a gram-negative, anaerobic, filamentous, obligate intracellular pathogenic clostridium. TD is often reported to be more frequent in foals (which are less than 45 days old and immunocompromised individuals), laboratory rabbits, mice, rats, and guinea pigs. Adult horses are generally found to be resistant to the infection. The fecal-oral route of transmission in foals is supported by successful experimental infection[24] and is more prevalent in young ones of mares older than 6 years suggesting a possible role for colostrum quality in disease development.[25] Predisposing factors in laboratory animals are immunosuppression, stress, high environmental temperatures, overcrowding, poor sanitation, changes in diet, and sulfonamide and corticosteroid administration.[26] The condition is also classified as a clostridial hepatitis based on the lesions associated with the infection. The mode of transmission is fecal-oral, with ingestion of spores from a fecal-contaminated environment by young animals. In affected animals, *C piliforme* proliferates in the intestinal mucosa, resulting in necrosis, and then disseminates to the liver and other organs. Virulence factors for this microorganism have not been identified, to date.[27,28]

Paeniclostridium sordellii

Paeniclostridium sordellii (previously *Clostridium sordellii*) has been frequently associated with gas gangrene in humans and several animal species, including horses. *Paeniclostridium sordellii* has been implicated in a myriad of sporadic infections in both humans and animals, which are characterized by a mild or completely absent inflammatory response. A common inhabitant of soil, the organism can also be found rarely in the intestinal content of clinically healthy animals.[29] *Paeniclostridium sordellii* is characterized as a Gram-positive, sporulating anaerobic rod that has been associated mainly with fatal toxic shock-like syndrome in humans,[30] gas gangrene in ruminants, pigs, and horses,[31] abomasitis in lambs, necrotic enteritis in chickens,[32] ulcerative enteritis in quail, omphalitis in foals,[33] and other histotoxic and enteric infections in wildlife, including bears and pelicans.[34] However, its role in enteric diseases of animals has not been fully determined. *Paeniclostridium sordellii*-associated enterocolitis in seven horses was reported recently[35] which had an inflammatory intestinal disease. They had lesions in both the small and large intestine characterized by segmental mucosal or transmural hemorrhages with mucosal erosions and ulcers, and diffuse pseudomembrane formation. The pathogen produces several toxins, although it is usually assumed that two of them, namely lethal toxin (TcsL) and hemorrhagic toxin (TcsH), are mainly responsible for the virulence of this microorganism.[36] The toxins of *P sordellii* are often compared with toxins A and B (TcdA and TcdB) of *C difficile*, and it has been reported that a specific antiserum against the lethal toxin of *P sordellii* successfully neutralized the cytotoxic and lethal activities of *C difficile* TcdB.[37,38]

EPIZOOTIOLOGY/ZOONOTIC POTENTIAL

Clostridioides difficile is considered a nosocomial pathogen associated with diarrhea and pseudomembranous colitis in hospitalized patients. First isolated in 1935, it is now recognized as a major cause of gastrointestinal disease affecting both animals and humans.[39] Disease in horses due to *C difficile* can cause discomfort in its mildest form and debilitating complications and death at its most severe and as they are used as performance, work, and companion animals, the zoonotic potential is increased. In addition, a significant association between proximity to livestock farms and the occurrence of community-acquired CDI case clusters and relatedness of strains isolated from paired pig and farmer samples were reported.[40,41] Though there are inconsistencies associated with the reported prevalence and impact of the disease in horses, 5% to 90% isolation rates of *C difficile* are observed in animals with diarrhea and acute colitis.[42,43] The greatest concern for humans is from the hypervirulent, ribotype 027/NAP1 strain, which has also been identified in horses[44] and ribotype 078, a strain that is common in food animals, is associated with CDI in humans.[45,46] This overlap of strains in humans and animals highlights the need for a One Health approach to understand and control the disease and underscores the need for veterinarians to be aware and proactive in biosecurity practices to mitigate disease risks for both humans and horses.[47,48]

CLINICAL SIGNS

The clinical presentation of clostridial diseases causing enterocolitis is similar to other causes of enterocolitis in horses and is not highly specific. Diarrhea and fever are the most common clinical signs observed alongside signs of colic. The appearance and progression of clinical signs can be peracute, acute or gradual in nature. In peracute cases, sudden death with or without clinical signs is observed. Although diarrhea without any systemic changes is encountered, inappetence, abdominal pain, colic, depression, pyrexia, and toxemia may also be present. Generally, in adult horses, extraintestinal symptoms are not frequent but in foals, meningitis, endocarditis, thrombosis, pneumonia, and arthritis are associated with clostridial infections.[49] In *C piliforme* infection, intestinal infection can spread to liver and other organs causing jaundice as a clinical manifestation.[50]

DIAGNOSIS

A presumptive diagnosis can be achieved by clinical signs, gross, and histological lesions in the animal. This can be further supported by the isolation of the pathogen from the intestinal contents. A history of antimicrobial therapy, in particular, and other procedures with potential for altering the gut microbiome, such as deworming and colic surgery, can be supportive in making accurate diagnosis. As many of the enteric clostridial organisms produce nonspecific clinical signs, differential diagnosis between species is important for human and animal welfare. Fecal screening by quantitative polymerase chain reaction (PCR) for Toxin A and B genes and detection of fecal toxins by enzyme-linked immunosorbent assay (ELISA) is useful in achieving a clinical diagnosis of *C difficile* diarrhea. Repeated screening may be necessary. Isolation of a large number of the organism and PCR toxinotyping of the isolates are also reported to be beneficial for CDAD diagnosis.[51] Similar diagnostic tools are reported to be useful in *C perfringens* infection, where culture and isolation followed by PCR genotyping to identify strain types is found to be of help in diagnosis. Specific PCR identification of enterotoxin, alpha, beta, epsilon and iota is supportive. Identification of specific toxin directly from feces using ELISA or reverse passive latex agglutination (RPLA) is another approach that has been adopted.[12] In TD, a presumptive diagnosis can be reached with clinical signs of acute focal or multifocal hepatocellular necrosis on necropsy. An antemortem diagnosis might be achieved; however, a fine-needle liver biopsy and PCR of the biopsy specimen(s) are required. Aggressive supportive care is required for a successful outcome.[52]

TREATMENT

Supportive therapy is most helpful in the treatment of enteric colitis in horses. Cessation of antimicrobial therapy if any, fluid therapy, and supportive nursing care are useful in the clinical management of colitis. If a causative organism is identified, targeted treatment with specific antimicrobial treatment is used by clinicians. Metronidazole is widely used to treat colitis, whereas vancomycin is another option for therapy.[53,54] In CDAD treatment metronidazole is still considered the primary line of treatment. As toxins play a major role in the clinical symptoms, toxin absorption using Di-tri-octahedral smectite is found to help in toxin absorption in colitis from *C difficile* and *C perfringens* toxins.[55] Though no studies strongly support their efficacy, commercially available probiotics can be used to attempt to control and prevent dysbiosis and diarrhea in equine colitis. Fecal microbiota transplantation is another therapy that may be beneficial in CDAD, but supportive studies in horses are very limited and the risk of transfer of other potential enteric pathogens, including rotavirus (especially in foals), and *Salmonella spp.* must be considered.

PREVENTION

Control of the suspected risk factors for the development of clostridial enteritis is the best available approach to the prevention of the disease, in the absence of objective information. As dysbiosis involving the disruption of the normal healthy intestinal flora is the predisposing cause, prudent and controlled use of antimicrobials, especially in higher risk patients, can be adopted. Sudden dietary changes, deworming, transportation, and other stress factors should be avoided or managed when known disturbances to the gut microbiome, such as during antibiotic usage, to ensure better gut health and disease prevention. Better hygiene, isolation of infected animals, and proper disposal of infected materials, including preventive steps adopted by personnel, will help in preventing the spread of infection to susceptible animals. Use of bleach and accelerated hydrogen peroxide with environmental biosecurity efforts have been found to limit the environmental spore load.

SUMMARY

The understanding of the pathogenesis of equine enteric clostridial organisms is an active, evolving field. Advances will improve our knowledge both from the animal welfare and human health perspectives. The zoonotic nature of this group of diseases makes them relevant in the age of One health, as a significant amount of close human-equine interactions occurs for business and pleasure. Economic and welfare reasons prompt a better understanding of enteric clostridial pathogenesis, treatment, and control of the infection in horses and ongoing efforts are needed to advance clinical outcomes.

CLINICS CARE POINTS

- Aggressive supportive care for clostridial enteric diseases is essential for a positive outcome, regardless of etiology.
- A complete history and physical examination are essential to direct treatment approaches while diagnostics are pending.
- A complete blood count (CBC) and serum biochemistry may be indicative of hepatic or bowel disease and aid in treatment decisions.
- Supportive care for equine colitis frequently requires immediate treatment for fluid deficits and electrolyte derangements. Means of neutralizing suspected toxins for enteric disease should be considered.
- Use of antibiotics to treat enteric clostridial diseases is often controversial; however, immediate treatment of suspected Tyzzer's disease with penicillin or other antibiotics is likely essential for a good outcome.

REFERENCES

1. McCollum DL, Rodriguez JM. Detection, treatment, and prevention of Clostridium difficile infection. Clin Gastroenterol Hepatol 2012;10(6):581–92.
2. Bartlett JG, Onderdonk AB, Cisneros RL, et al. Clindamycin-associated colitis due to a toxin-producing species of Clostridium in hamsters. J Infect Dis 1977; 136(5):701–5.
3. Båverud V. Clostridium difficile infections in animals with special reference to the horse. A review. Vet Q 2002;24(4):203–19.
4. Båverud V. Clostridium difficile diarrhea: infection control in horses. Vet Clin Equine Pract 2004a;20(3):615–30.

5. Centers for Disease Control and Prevention (CDC). Surveillance for community-associated Clostridium difficile–Connecticut, 2006. MMWR.Morbidity Mortality Weekly Rep 2008;57(13):340–3.

6. Freeman J, Bauer M, Baines SD, et al. The changing epidemiology of Clostridium difficile infections. Clin Microbiol Rev 2010;23(3):529–49.

7. Schoster A, Staempfli HR, Arroyo LG, et al. Longitudinal study of Clostridium difficile and antimicrobial susceptibility of Escherichia coli in healthy horses in a community setting. Vet Microbiol 2011;159(3–4):364–70.

8. Artiushin S, Timoney J, Fettinger M, et al. Immunisation of mares with binding domains of toxins A and B of C lostridium difficile elicits serum and colostral antibodies that block toxin binding. Equine Vet J 2013;45(4):476–80.

9. Davies AH, Roberts AK, Shone CC, et al. Super toxins from a super bug: structure and function of Clostridium difficile toxins. Biochem J 2011;436(3):517–26.

10. Keel MK, Songer J. The comparative pathology of Clostridium difficile-associated disease. Vet Pathol 2006;43(3):225–40.

11. Uzal FA, Arroyo LG, Navarro MA, et al. Bacterial and viral enterocolitis in horses: a review. J Vet Diagn Invest 2022;34(3):354–75.

12. Weese J, Staempfli H, Prescott J. A prospective study of the roles of Clostridium difficile and enterotoxigenic Clostridium perfringens in equine diarrhoea. Equine Vet J 2001a;33(4):403–9.

13. Diab SS, Kinde H, Moore J, et al. Pathology of Clostridium perfringens type C enterotoxemia in horses. Vet Pathol 2012;49(2):255–63.

14. Bueschel D, Walker R, Woods L, et al. Enterotoxigenic Clostridium perfringens type A necrotic enteritis in a foal. J Am Vet Med Assoc 1998;213(9):1305–7, 1280.

15. Donaldson MT, Palmer JE. Prevalence of Clostridium perfringens enterotoxin and Clostridium difficile toxin A in feces of horses with diarrhea and colic. J Am Vet Med Assoc 1999;215(3):358–61.

16. East LM, Dargatz DA, Traub-Dargatz JL, et al. Foaling-management practices associated with the occurrence of enterocolitis attributed to Clostridium perfringens infection in the equine neonate. Prev Vet Med 2000;46(1):61–74.

17. Fernandez-Miyakawa ME, Fisher DJ, Poon R, et al. Both epsilon-toxin and beta-toxin are important for the lethal properties of Clostridium perfringens type B isolates in the mouse intravenous injection model. Infect Immun 2007;75(3):1443–52.

18. Netherwood T, Wood J, Mumford J, et al. Molecular analysis of the virulence determinants ofClostridium perfringens associated with foal diarrhoea. Vet J 1998;155(3):289–94.

19. Tillotson K, Traub-Dargatz JL, Dickinson CE, et al. Population-based study of fecal shedding of Clostridium perfringens in broodmares and foals. J Am Vet Med Assoc 2002;220(3):342–8.

20. Uzal FA, Songer JG, Prescott JF, et al. Clostridial diseases of animals. Hoboken (NJ): John Wiley & Sons; 2016.

21. Gohari IM, Parreira V, Timoney J, et al. NetF-positive Clostridium perfringens in neonatal foal necrotising enteritis in Kentucky. Vet Rec 2016;178(9):216.

22. Gohari IM, Parreira VR, Nowell VJ, et al. A novel pore-forming toxin in type A Clostridium perfringens is associated with both fatal canine hemorrhagic gastroenteritis and fatal foal necrotizing enterocolitis. PLoS ONE 2015;10(4):e0122684.

23. Mehdizadeh Gohari I, Unterer S, Whitehead AE, et al. NetF-producing Clostridium perfringens and its associated diseases in dogs and foals. J Vet Diagn Invest 2020;32(2):230–8.

24. Swerczek TW. Tyzzer's disease in foals: retrospective studies from 1969 to 2010. Can Vet J = La revue Veterinaire Canadienne 2013;54(9):876–80.
25. Fosgate GT, Hird DW, Read DH, et al. Risk factors for Clostridium piliforme infection in foals. J Am Vet Med Assoc 2002;220(6):785–90.
26. Ikegami T, Shirota K, Une Y, et al. Naturally occurring Tyzzer's disease in a calf. Vet Pathol 1999;36(3):253–5.
27. Barthold SW, Griffey SM, Percy DH. Pathology of laboratory rodents and rabbits. Hoboken (NJ): John Wiley & Sons; 1991.
28. Navarro MA, Uzal FA. Pathobiology and diagnosis of clostridial hepatitis in animals. J Vet Diagn Invest 2020;32(2):192–202.
29. Benavides J, González L, Dagleish M, et al. Diagnostic pathology in microbial diseases of sheep or goats. Vet Microbiol 2015;181(1–2):15–26.
30. Zane S, Guarner J. Gynecologic clostridial toxic shock in women of reproductive age. Curr Infect Dis Rep 2011;13(6):561–70.
31. Simpson KM, Callan RJ, Van Metre DC. "Clostridial Abomasitis and Enteritis in Ruminants", The Veterinary clinics of North America. Food Anim Pract 2018;34(1): 155–84.
32. Rimoldi G, Uzal F, Chin RP, et al. Necrotic enteritis in chickens associated with Clostridium sordellii. Avian Dis 2015;59(3):447–51.
33. Ortega J, Daft B, Assis R, et al. Infection of internal umbilical remnant in foals by Clostridium sordellii. Vet Pathol 2007;44(3):269–75.
34. Lueders I, Ludwig C, Kasberg J, et al. Unusual outbreak of fatal clostridiosis in a group of captive brown pelicans (Pelecanus occidentalis). J Avian Med Surg 2017;31(4):359–63.
35. Nyaoke AC, Navarro MA, Fresneda K, et al. Paeniclostridium (Clostridium) sordellii–associated enterocolitis in 7 horses. J Vet Diagn Invest 2020;32(2): 239–45.
36. Vidor C, Awad M, Lyras D. Antibiotic resistance, virulence factors and genetics of Clostridium sordellii. Res Microbiol 2015;166(4):368–74.
37. Popoff MR. Clostridium difficile and Clostridium sordellii toxins, proinflammatory versus anti-inflammatory response. Toxicon 2018;149:54–64.
38. Unger-Torroledo L, Straub R, Lehmann AD, et al. Lethal toxin of Clostridium sordellii is associated with fatal equine atypical myopathy. Vet Microbiol 2010; 144(3–4):487–92.
39. Lim SC, Knight D, Riley TV. Clostridium difficile and one health. Clin Microbiol Infect 2020;26(7):857–63.
40. Anderson DJ, Rojas LF, Watson S, et al. Identification of novel risk factors for community-acquired Clostridium difficile infection using spatial statistics and geographic information system analyses. PLoS One 2017;12(5):e0176285.
41. Knight DR, Riley TV. Genomic delineation of zoonotic origins of Clostridium difficile. Front Public Health 2019;7:164.
42. Frederick J, Giguere S, Sanchez L. Infectious agents detected in the feces of diarrheic foals: a retrospective study of 233 cases (2003–2008). J Vet Intern Med 2009;23(6):1254–60.
43. Thean S, Elliott B, Riley TV. Clostridium difficile in horses in Australia–a preliminary study. J Med Microbiol 2011;60(8):1188–92.
44. Gerding DN. Global epidemiology of Clostridium difficile infection in 2010. Infect Control Hosp Epidemiol 2010;31(S1):S32–4.
45. Medina-Torres CE, Weese JS, Staempfli HR. Prevalence of Clostridium difficile in horses. Vet Microbiol 2011;152(1–2):212–5.

46. Weese JS, Wakeford T, Reid-Smith R, et al. Longitudinal investigation of Clostridium difficile shedding in piglets. Anaerobe 2010;16(5):501–4.
47. Hain-Saunders NM, Knight DR, Bruce M, et al. Clostridioides difficile infection and One Health: an equine perspective. Environ Microbiol 2022;24(3):985–97.
48. Rodriguez C, Taminiau B, Broeck JV, et al. Clostridium difficile in food and animals: a comprehensive review. Adv Microbiol Infect Dis Public Health 2016;65–92.
49. Ruby R, Magdesian KG, Kass PH. Comparison of clinical, microbiologic, and clinicopathologic findings in horses positive and negative for Clostridium difficile infection. J Am Vet Med Assoc 2009;234(6):777–84.
50. Sweeney HJ, Greig A. Infectious necrotic hepatitis in a horse. Equine Vet J 1986; 18(2):150–1.
51. Madewell BR, Tang YJ, Jang S, et al. Apparent outbreaks of Clostridium difficile-associated diarrhea in horses in a veterinary medical teaching hospital. J Vet Diagn Invest 1995;7(3):343–6.
52. Borchers A, Magdesian KG, Halland S, et al. Successful treatment and polymerase chain reaction (PCR) confirmation of Tyzzer's disease in a foal and clinical and pathologic characteristics of 6 additional foals (1986-2005). J Vet Intern Med 2006;20(5):1212–8.
53. Musher DM, Aslam S, Logan N, et al. Relatively poor outcome after treatment of Clostridium difficile colitis with metronidazole. Clin Infect Dis 2005;40(11): 1586–90.
54. Pépin J, Valiquette L, Gagnon S, et al. Outcomes of Clostridium difficile-associated disease treated with metronidazole or vancomycin before and after the emergence of NAP1/027. Am Coll Gastroenterol ACG 2007;102(12):2781–8.
55. Lawler JB, Hassel DM, Magnuson RJ, et al. Adsorptive effects of di-tri-octahedral smectite on Clostridium perfringens alpha, beta, and beta-2 exotoxins and equine colostral antibodies. Am J Vet Res 2008;69(2):233–9.

Salmonella in Horses

Brandy A. Burgess, DVM, MSc, PhD

KEYWORDS

- Salmonellosis • Equine • Diagnostic testing • Shedding

KEY POINTS (CLINICS CARE POINTS)

- Horses with systemic illness—regardless of body system affected—and those having any one of the classic triad of clinical signs (fever, diarrhea, or leukopenia) have a higher likelihood of shedding.
- Horses can intermittently shed low levels of organisms necessitating the testing of multiple samples (eg, 3–5) using enriched culture methods to improve the overall sensitivity of the testing strategy.
- Early risk recognition and implementation of prevention efforts are critical to the effective management of equine populations and their environments.

INTRODUCTION AND BACKGROUND
What Is It?

The genus *Salmonella* consists of 2 species, *Salmonella enterica* and *Salmonella bongori*, with *S enterica* being subdivided into 6 subspecies (*enterica, salamae, arizonae, diarizonae, houtenae,* and *indica*). Collectively, there are more than 2400 serovars (often referred to as serotypes) that differ by surface O-antigens (polysaccharide portion of lipopolysaccharide) and H-antigens (filamentous portion of flagella or flagellin). As a member of the family Enterobacteriaceae, *S enterica* is a gram-negative facultative anaerobic bacterium that colonizes the small intestine, cecum, and colon of cold-blooded and warm-blooded vertebrates. This review will focus on *S enterica* subspecies Enterica, which accounts for approximately 59% of all serovars and an estimated 99% of infections in warm-blooded animals.[1,2]

A few definitions

In the literature, animals with detectable *Salmonella* are commonly classified as having clinical disease or subclinical infection. Generally, *clinical disease* is an acute or chronic gastrointestinal disease or sepsis, whereas *subclinical infection* is the detection of organism in a healthy animal (ie, without clinical signs). Animals with subclinical infections are often referred to as subclinical carriers or asymptomatic shedders, or to

Department of Population Health, College of Veterinary Medicine, University of Georgia, 2200 College Station Road, Athens, GA 30602, USA
E-mail address: brandy.burgess@uga.edu

Vet Clin Equine 39 (2023) 25–35
https://doi.org/10.1016/j.cveq.2022.11.005
0749-0739/23/© 2022 Elsevier Inc. All rights reserved.

have subclinical colonization. For simplicity, this review will categorize *Salmonella* infections as clinical disease or subclinical infection.

Natural history of disease

S enterica transmission occurs by the fecal–oral route and can result in enterocolitis, often manifesting with diarrhea, bacteremia, or subclinical infection. Generally considered an opportunistic pathogen, it is more likely to cause clinical disease with high exposure (ie, high infective dose) or among patients with an increased susceptibility (eg, neonates and patients with severe systemic illness), and often depends on the infecting serovar. Although the equine practitioner tends to focus on clinically affected animals, subclinical infection and shedding in the absence of disease is likely much more common.[3] *S enterica* can present a diagnostic challenge as horses tend to shed intermittently and at low levels, necessitating testing of multiple samples and enriched culture methods to improve the overall sensitivity of the testing strategy.

Why Is It Important?

S enterica is one of the most commonly identified agents associated with epidemic disease in veterinary hospitals[4] and is frequently associated with on-farm contamination.[5] As subclinical infection and shedding is much more common than clinical infections, when *Salmonella* spreads among patients, environmental contamination is predictably present and can become widespread before the scope of the problem is realized.[3,6–9] Oftentimes, these outbreaks result in significant morbidity and mortality, pose a clear risk to veterinary patients and personnel, and come with great financial costs.[6,10]

Why Should We Care?

Veterinary practitioners have both an ethical and a legal obligation to appropriately manage risks related to infectious diseases, such as salmonellosis, in animal populations and their environments. The veterinarian's oath calls attention to a veterinarian's ethical obligation to protect the individual patient *(relief of animal suffering)*, protect the animal population of the present and the future *(protection of animal health and welfare)*, and to protect people *(promotion of public health)*.[11] The General Duty Clause, 5(a) (1), of the Occupational Safety and Health Act of 1970, highlights an employer's legal obligation to provide a workplace that is free from recognized hazards that are likely to result in "serious physical harm."[12] Although veterinary infection control is in its early stages, there is a developing recognizable standard of practice; due effort must be given to the prevention of infectious disease transmission within animal populations and facilities.[13] In fact, a survey conducted in 2004 among North American veterinary teaching hospitals found that all 30 survey respondents had some form of infection control program in their equine hospitals, as did some of the more progressive private veterinary hospitals.[4]

EPIDEMIOLOGY IN HORSES

Nosocomial outbreaks of salmonellosis have been repeatedly shown to be a constant risk in all types of veterinary hospitals, resulting in significant morbidity and mortality among hospitalized patients and zoonotic infections in personnel.[6–8,14,15]

Prevalence of Salmonella Shedding

Shedding prevalence of *S enterica* can vary markedly with health status, season of the year, and geographic region. Among *healthy* horses in the general equine population, shedding prevalence is an estimated 0.8% (SE 0.5)[5] and can range from 0.5% to 7%

among *hospitalized* horses when tested on admission or throughout hospitalization, respectively.[5,16–18] *Seasonality* of shedding is a consistent finding with a higher prevalence in late summer and early fall and a lower prevalence in the springtime.[5,17,19–21] *Geographic region* may also influence shedding with warmer and wetter regions of North America having a higher reported prevalence compared with cooler and dryer regions.[5]

Risk Factors for Salmonella Shedding

The central tenet of epidemiology tells us that disease does not occur randomly in populations. Rather, there are key factors related to the agent, host, and environment (ie, the epidemiologic triad) that contribute to the development of disease.

The agent

As with any other infectious disease, agent characteristics of *Salmonella* likely play a role in the occurrence of disease including the infecting serovar, the inoculating dose, and environmental persistence. Time to shedding varies by infecting *serotype*, ranging from approximately 1 to 5 days among naturally infected horses.[21,22] That being said, this is likely confounded by health status and infectious dose with increased susceptibility and higher infectious doses being at the lower end of this range. A meta-analysis of 43 studies experimentally inoculating healthy animals (horses, cattle, sheep), found that on average, shedding occurred within 1.3 days (95% CI 1.22, 1.39; range 0.75–3 days).[23] It is important to note that inoculating doses were higher than expected in natural infection ranging from 10^4 to 10^{13}. Therefore, the average time to shedding reported is likely shorter than what would be expected in natural infections. *Salmonella* organisms can persist in damp environments that contain organic debris, forming biofilms, and environmental reservoirs that serve as potential sources for continued transmission.[24]

The host

Historically, we consider a triad of clinical signs—diarrhea, fever, and leukopenia—to be indicating *Salmonella* shedding among horses.[25,26] A meta-analysis of 43 studies experimentally inoculating healthy animals (horses, cattle, sheep), found that on average, pyrexia occurred within 1.5 days of infection (95% CI 1.47, 1.55) and diarrhea occurred within 1.7 days of infection (95% CI 1.62, 1.83).[23] Note that inoculating doses ranged from 10^4 to 10^{13}, higher than expected in natural infection, and therefore, the average days reported are likely fewer than what would be expected in natural infections. Interestingly, this study also reported an average time to shedding of 1.3 days (95% CI 1.22, 1.39) suggesting that by the time fever and/or diarrhea are recognized, animals are likely to already be shedding *Salmonella* in their feces.[23] Although more contemporary studies continue to support this observation,[27–29] this triad of clinical signs can occur rather infrequently, only accounting for an estimated 2.7% of shedding among a hospital population (ie, the population attributable fraction).[20] Indeed, an estimated 70% of shedding can be attributed to systemic illness, irrespective of the body system affected, with more severe disease having a higher shedding probability.[20]

Although the idea that horses with more severe disease are more likely to shed makes biological sense, it is important to note that during the years, this has not been a consistent finding. Many studies have evaluated shedding risk among horses with gastrointestinal disease, and some studies have reported an increased risk associated with abdominal surgery or with vascular compromising conditions,[8,9,21,22,27,30] whereas other studies have not found similar associations.[9,31,32] That being said, with an estimated shedding prevalence ranging from 4.3% up to 13%, horses with gastro-intestinal disease or colic are often managed separately from the general patient population at many equine facilities.[16,21,32]

Many reports suggest that antimicrobial therapy affects the probability of *Salmonella* shedding; however, this too has been inconsistent.[9,21,29,31–33] One subgroup that is consistently reported to be more likely to shed *Salmonella* during hospitalization are those admitted to critical care units.[34] Horses in this subgroup likely have more severe disease as well as susceptibility, and of particular concern are critically ill foals with gastrointestinal disease that require intensive management.[21]

Although horses with severe disease are likely to be more susceptible to infection, they are also more likely to be tested. As such, extrapolating findings from studies of limited patient populations, for example, animals involved in outbreaks, should be done with caution. Studies reporting the occurrence of endemic disease among the general horse population have found that both patient and hospital factors may be important, including transportation distance (travel time >1 hour), abnormal findings on nasogastric intubation, diarrhea, leukopenia ($\leq$5000 WBC/μL), previous antimicrobial therapy, abdominal surgery, and duration of hospitalization.[16–18,20,21,27,32,33] In contrast, being admitted for an elective procedure, such as musculoskeletal disease or cryptorchidism, or being a hospital companion, tends to decrease the likelihood for shedding.[16]

One of the challenges in managing salmonellosis in horses is the potential influence of shedding on the positive-horse and its stablemates. Currently, there are limited data on the duration of shedding, and therefore, the period of time a shedding horse may need to be managed differently. An early conference report suggested positive-horses may shed for up to 30 days; however, the study population was very limited, reducing the generalizability this finding.[35] A more recent prospective study, which tested positive-horses weekly, preliminarily found an estimated median shedding duration of 54 days (range 14–121 days) and 31 days (range 4–138 days) among horses with clinical disease and subclinical infection, respectively.[36] This study also found that, on average, horses with severe disease tended to shed for longer, as did horses receiving oral antimicrobials. With this in mind, it is likely prudent to take precautions when managing these horses for 6 to 8 weeks. Indeed, it has been shown that when these horses return to their home farms, they do not seem to adversely affect stablemates as long as precautions are in place.[29,37]

The environment

Disseminated environmental contamination is a universal feature associated with ongoing *Salmonella* transmission within a facility.[6–8] Common contributing factors include suboptimal environmental hygiene practices such as ineffective infection control policies, damaged floor surfaces that promote the accumulation of contamination, and use of porous, noncleanable surfaces such as unsealed concrete and wood[6,8,15]; and contamination of common use equipment such as buckets, nasogastric tubes, and rectal thermometers.[8,9,15] Additionally, the probability of detecting *Salmonella* in the environment increases as demand on personnel increases (eg, periods of high case load or times of limited personnel).[20] Although this review is focusing on horses and their environments, species or management circumstances may be important factors as intensively managed cattle are more likely to shed than horses, an important element when managing horses in a multispecies facility.[20] Additionally, a seasonal occurrence to shedding is consistently reported with it being highest in late summer and early fall, and lowest in the spring,[5,17,19–21] although this may also be influenced by geographic location with warmer and wetter regions having a higher reported prevalence compared with cooler and dryer ones.[5]

DIAGNOSTIC TESTING AND TEST INTERPRETATION

Detection of *S enterica* in horses can present a diagnostic challenge due to the intermittent nature and low level of organisms shed in equine feces. As a result, irrespective of analytical sensitivity of the testing methods (eg, enriched culture, polymerase chain reaction [PCR], lateral flow immunoassays [LFIs]), the overall detection system (ie, sample type combined with sample processing and detection method) will have a poorer epidemiologic sensitivity (ie, lower probability of detecting truly shedding horses). To some degree, this may be overcome by testing larger sample volumes,[38] using enriched culture methodologies, and testing multiple samples from the same animal.[21] The general recommendation is to test 3 to 5 enriched-cultures, obtained in a short time frame (ie, sampling at 12–24 hour intervals). Assuming independence of test results, the estimated sensitivity when interpreting in parallel is 44% for a single culture, 66% for 2 cultures, 82% for 3 cultures, and 97% for 5 cultures.[35] With this in mind, practitioners can have reasonable confidence that a horse is truly negative with 3 to 5 negative cultures. It is important to recognize that regardless of detection method, it should be validated and optimized for its intended use (ie, equine fecal and environmental samples). In the case of *S enterica*, many different *Salmonella* serovars can cause disease and the distribution can change over time.[19,39] Therefore, knowledge of the common serovars in a given practice location is important to ensure accurate detection.[40]

Practitioners should be aware of the testing methods available, their associated strengths and limitations, and know which method a laboratory is using because this can affect test sensitivity/specificity and ultimately its interpretations relative to disease control efforts.[39–42]

Culture of Fecal Samples

Detection of *S enterica* by bacterial culture can be affected by the type of sample (feces, swab, or rectal biopsy), distribution of target organism in the sample, sample weight or volume, intermittent shedding, culture media and method used, and laboratory proficiency.

Type of sample and sample storage

In general, culture of a rectal mucosal sample is more sensitive than a fecal culture, which is more sensitive than a rectal swab.[38,43] However, the invasive nature of obtaining a rectal mucosal sample may preclude its routine use. These differences may be attributed to the amount of material that is cultured as larger sample mass generally provides higher test sensitivity[38] and are affected by the culture media and method used.[44–46] Best practice is to refrigerate samples until processing as soon after collection as possible. That being said, organism recovery does not seem to be greatly impaired if processed the same day, after 6 days of refrigeration (4°C), or after 14 days of freezing (−15°C).[26]

Heterogeneity of organism in the sample

Salmonella organisms tend to cluster within a fecal sample (ie, are not homogenously distributed)[47] resulting in a greater likelihood that a single sample may not contain any organisms. As such, testing a small aliquot such as a rectal swab or less than 1 g or not thoroughly mixing the sample may result in a false-negative test result.

Sample weight or volume

In general, the larger the sample, the greater the sensitivity. This means that the relative sensitivity of culture increases with increasing sample weight,[38] which can be further improved by thoroughly mixing the sample to homogenously distribute organisms.[47]

Intermittent shedding

In horses, *Salmonella* organisms are intermittently shed at low numbers,[17,36,48] which affects the accuracy of detection methods when applied in practice. As such, we tend to test multiple samples (eg, 3–5 samples at 12–24-hour intervals) from the same animal[21] and use enriched culture methodologies, respectively.

Culture media and method

There are many different aerobic culture methods for the detection of *S enterica* that use a variety of broth and solid culture media, and incubation times and temperatures.[13–16,24,25] Each methodological choice leads to differences in test accuracy. For example, the analytical sensitivity of equine fecal culture has been reported to be as few as 4 cfu/g of feces when enriched in tetrathionate (TET) broth[44] and 100 cfu/g of feces when enriched in selenite broth.[45]

In general, using a *Salmonella* selective media (eg, TET, Rappaport-Vassiliadis) in an enrichment step will improve test sensitivity because it allows *Salmonella* organisms to grow while inhibiting the growth of competing bacteria.[46] Sensitivity can be further improved if plated on a selective media (eg, xylose-lysine-tergitol 4 or Hektoen enteric agar).[46]

Samples with low bacterial burdens, such as environmental samples, may benefit from preenrichment with nonselective media (eg, buffered peptone water [BPW]) because it allows for bacteria that may have been damaged due to environmental conditions to recover. Preenrichment is not recommended for samples containing high bacterial burdens such as fecal samples because competing bacteria may overgrow resulting in a false-negative test result.

Laboratory proficiency

The ability to detect *Salmonella* can vary greatly among laboratories. These differences are likely related to the use of less optimal culture methods such as harsh enrichment media or lower temperatures[39–42,46,49] or may simply be due to lower recovery rates when using the same methods.[41,50] With this in mind, it is important for practitioners to request confirmation of proficiency testing when selecting a laboratory.

Culture of environmental samples

Salmonella organisms are relatively hardy in damp environments that contain organic debris and can develop biofilms resulting in environmental reservoirs for infection. When sampling the hospital environment, electrostatic dust wipes are more sensitive than sterile sponges.[6,51,52] As with fecal culture, these differences may be attributed to the amount of material that is cultured (a function of the device used and surface area sampled) as larger sample generally provides higher test sensitivity[38] and the culture media and method used as indicated above. It is generally recommended to perform a preenrichment step in a nutrient rich media (eg, BPW) before performing an enriched culture. This allows organisms that may have been damaged or "injured" due to environmental conditions (eg, UV light, drying, exposure to disinfectants) to repair themselves before being exposed to relative harsh enrichment media. This will delay time to obtaining results but will improve overall test sensitivity.

Polymerase chain reaction

PCR is generally considered to be sensitive and specific for the detection of *Salmonella*.[53] The analytical sensitivity for PCR assays has been reported to be 100 cfu/g of equine feces when testing enriched cultures or 1000 cfu/g of feces when testing nonenriched samples. Using primers that target highly conserved genes ensures high analytical specificity because these assays can detect many serovars without cross-reacting with other common bacteria.[54] Although PCR assays are generally more rapid than enriched culture, providing results in 1 to 2 days compared with 2 to 5 days for enriched cultures,[45,54–56] its epidemiologic sensitivity is similarly limited due to low level, intermittent shedding of organisms. One consideration when using PCR is the fact that this assay can detect nonviable organisms as well as degraded DNA. As such, a positive test may not indicate an infectious risk. This may be important relative to its use for the detection of *Salmonella* in environmental samples because disinfectants target different parts of bacterial organisms. For example, quaternary ammonium and phenolic disinfectants target cytoplasmic membranes, leaving DNA intact, whereas bleach and formaldehyde degrade DNA. This could theoretically lead to differential detection rates when comparing PCR and culture methodologies.[57]

Lateral flow immunoassays
Commercially available LFIs, developed for use in food safety applications, may be a practical alternative to traditional detection methods for the detection of *Salmonella* in horses and their environments. Experimentally, it has been shown to have an analytical sensitivity of ~ 4 cfu/g of equine feces from enriched cultures, good analytical specificity detecting many different serovars, and can reliably detect organisms in 1-g samples after 18 hours in enriched cultures.[44,58,59] It is important to submit LFI-positive samples for follow-up culture to allow for further characterization of isolates (eg, serogroup, serotype, antimicrobial susceptibility) to aid in the assessment of transmission risks.

SUMMARY

Salmonella can be challenging to manage in horse populations. Clinical outcomes can range from mild diarrhea to severe disease, septicemia, and death. Horses are commonly subclinically infected and can intermittently shed for extended periods. As a result, the ability to detect positive-horses (ie, test sensitivity) is greatly affected and necessitates taking multiple samples during a short time period. Unfortunately, this delay in the detection typically leads to widespread environmental contamination, a common feature during outbreaks. Indeed, environmental isolates are commonly phenotypically similar (ie, serotype and antimicrobial susceptibility) to patient isolates, suggesting horses are a likely source for this contamination.[6,7,52,60] This observation emphasizes the importance of managing high risk groups, such as those animals with severe disease, to reduce the potential for contamination and transmission and to continue these precautions on positive-horses even when they return to their home farm. In doing so, veterinarians can reduce the risk of *Salmonella* to stablemates and their caretakers.

DISCLOSURE

The author has nothing to disclose.

REFERENCES

1. Lan R, Reeves PR, Octavia S. Population structure, origins and evolution of major *Salmonella enterica* clones. Infect Genet Evol 2009;9(5):996–1005.

2. Brenner FW, Villar RG, Angulo FJ, et al. Salmonella nomenclature. J Clin Microbiol 2000;38(7):2465–7.

3. Palmer JP, Benson CE, Whitlock RH. Subclinical salmonellosis in horses with colic. In: Equine colic research symposium. 1982. Athens, GA.

4. Benedict KM, Morley PS, Van Metre DC. Characteristics of biosecurity and infection control programs at veterinary teaching hospitals. J Am Vet Med Assoc 2008; 233(5):767–73.

5. Traub-Dargatz JL, Garber LP, Dedorka-Cray PJ, et al. Fecal shedding of Salmonella spp by horses in the United States during 1998 and 1999 and detection of Salmonella spp in grain and concentrate sources on equine operations. J Am Vet Med Assoc 2000;217(2):226–30.

6. Dallap Schaer BL, Aceto H, Rankin SC. Outbreak of salmonellosis caused by Salmonella enterica serovar Newport MDR-AmpC in a large animal veterinary teaching hospital. J Vet Intern Med 2010;24(5):1138–46.

7. Steneroden KK, Van Metre DC, Jackson C, et al. Detection and control of a nosocomial outbreak caused by Salmonella newport at a large animal hospital. J Vet Intern Med 2010;24(3):606–16.

8. Tillotson K, Savage CJ, Salman MD, et al. Outbreak of Salmonella infantis infection in a large animal veterinary teaching hospital. J Am Vet Med Assoc 1997; 211(12):1554–7.

9. Hird DW, Pappaioanou M, Smith BP. Case-control study of risk factors associated with isolation of Salmonella saintpaul in hospitalized horses. Am J Epidemiol 1984;120(6):852–64.

10. Weaver DR, Newman LS, Lezotte DD, et al. Perceptions regarding workplace hazards at a veterinary teaching hospital. J Am Vet Med Assoc 2010;237(1): 93–100.

11. Anonymous. Who we are: Veteriarian's oath. 2012 [cited 2012 January 1]; Available from: http://www.avma.org/about_avma/whoweare/oath.asp.

12. Morey RS. The Gereal Duty Clause of the Occupational Safety and Health Act of 1970. Harv Law Rev 1973;86(6):988–1005.

13. Morley P, Anderson M, Burgess B. Report of the third Havemeyer workshop on infection control in equine populations. Equine Vet J 2013;45(2).

14. Wright J, Tengelsen L, Smith K, et al. Multidrug-resistant Salmonella Typhimurium in four animal facilities. Emerg Infect Dis 2005;11(8):1235–41.

15. Schott HC 2nd, Ewart SL, Walker RD, et al. An outbreak of salmonellosis among horses at a veterinary teaching hospital. J Am Vet Med Assoc 2001;218(7): 1152–9.

16. Alinovi CA, Ward MP, Couetil LL, et al. Risk factors for fecal shedding of Salmonella from horses in a veterinary teaching hospital. Prev Vet Med 2003;60(4): 307–17.

17. Smith BP, Reina-Guerra M, Hardy AJ. Prevalence and epizootiology of equine salmonellosis. J Am Vet Med Assoc 1978;172(3):353–6.

18. Traub-Dargatz JL, Salman MD, Jones RL. Epidemiologic study of salmonellae shedding in the feces of horses and potential risk factors for development of the infection in hospitalized horses. J Am Vet Med Assoc 1990;196(10):1617–22.

19. Carter JD, Hird DW, Farver TB, et al. Salmonellosis in hospitalized horses: seasonality and case fatality rates. J Am Vet Med Assoc 1986;188(2):163–7.

20. Burgess BA, Morley PS. Risk factors for shedding of Salmonella enterica among hospitalized large animals over a 10-year period in a veterinary teaching hospital. J Vet Intern Med 2019;33(5):2239–48.

21. Ernst NS, Colahan PT, Giguere S, et al. Risk factors associated with fecal Salmonella shedding among hospitalized horses with signs of gastrointestinal tract disease. J Am Vet Med Assoc 2004;225(2):275–81.

22. House JK, House AM, Kamiya DY, et al. Risk factors for nosocomial Salmonella infection among hospitalized horses. J Am Vet Med Assoc 1999;214(10):1511–6.
23. Aceto H, Miller SA, Smith G. Onset of diarrhea and pyrexia and time to detection of Salmonella enterica subsp enterica in feces in experimental studies of cattle, horses, goats, and sheep after infection per os. J Am Vet Med Assoc 2011; 238(10):1333–9.
24. Shatila F, Yasa I, Yalcin HT. Biofilm Formation by Salmonella enterica Strains. Curr Microbiol 2021;78(4):1150–8.
25. Dorn CR, Coffman JR, Schmidt DA, et al. Neutropenia and salmonellosis in hospitalized horses. J Am Vet Med Assoc 1975;166(1):65–7.
26. Owen R, Fullerton JN, Tizard IR, et al. Studies on experimental enteric salmonellosis in ponies. Can J Comp Med 1979;43(3):247–54.
27. Dallap Schaer BL, Aceto H, Caruso MA, et al. Identification of predictors of Salmonella shedding in adult horses presented for acute colic. J Vet Intern Med 2012;26(5):1177–85.
28. Southwood LL, Lindborg S, Aceto HW. Influence of Salmonella status on the long-term outcome of horses after colic surgery. *Vet Surg* 2017;46(6):780–8.
29. Burgess BA, Bauknecht K, Slovis NM, et al. Factors associated with equine shedding of multi-drug-resistant Salmonella enterica and its impact on health outcomes. Equine Vet J 2018;50(5):616–23.
30. Ekiri AB, Mackay RJ, Gaskin JM, et al. Epidemiologic analysis of nosocomial Salmonella infections in hospitalized horses. *J Am Vet Med Assoc* 2009;234(1): 108–19.
31. Hird DW, Casebolt DB, Carter JD, et al. Risk factors for salmonellosis in hospitalized horses. *J Am Vet Med Assoc* 1986;188(2):173–7.
32. Kim LM, Morley PS, Traub-Dargatz JL, et al. Factors associated with Salmonella shedding among equine colic patients at a veterinary teaching hospital. *J Am Vet Med Assoc* 2001;218(5):740–8.
33. Dunowska M, Patterson G, Traub-Dargatz JL, et al. Recent progress in controlling Salmonella in Veterinry Hospitals. In: 50th annual convention of the American association of equine practitioners. 2004. Lexington, KY.
34. Mainar-Jaime RC, House AM, Kamiya DY, et al. Influence of fecal shedding of Salmonella organisms on mortality in hospitalized horses. *J Am Vet Med Assoc* 1998; 213(8):1162–6.
35. Palmer JE, Benson CE. Salmonella shedding in the equine. In: International symposium on Salmonella. 1984. New Orleans, LA.
36. Burgess BA, Aceto H, Barrell EA, et al. ACVIM Forum Research Report Program. J Vet Intern Med 2019;33(5):2359.
37. Hartnack AK, Van Metre DC, Morley PS. Salmonella enterica shedding in hospitalized horses and associations with diarrhea occurrence among their stablemates and gastrointestinal-related illness or death following discharge. J Am Vet Med Assoc 2012;240(6):726–33.
38. Funk JA, Davies PR, Nichols MA. The effect of fecal sample weight on detection of Salmonella enterica in swine feces. J Vet Diagn Invest 2000;12(5):412–8.
39. Singer RS, Isaacson RE, Hanson TE, et al. Do microbial interactions and cultivation media decrease the accuracy of Salmonella surveillance systems and outbreak investigations? *J Food Prot* 2009;72(4):707–13.
40. Rostagno MH, Gailey JK, Hurd HS, et al. Culture methods differ on the isolation of Salmonella enterica serotypes from naturally contaminated swine fecal samples. J Vet Diagn Invest 2005;17(1):80–3.

41. Voogt N, Nagelkerke NJ, van de Giessen AW, et al. Differences between reference laboratories of the European community in their ability to detect Salmonella species. Eur J Clin Microbiol Infect Dis 2002;21(6):449–54.

42. Love BC, Rostagno MH. Comparison of five culture methods for Salmonella isolation from swine fecal samples of known infection status. J Vet Diagn Invest 2008; 20(5):620–4.

43. Palmer JE, Morris DD, Acland HM, et al. Comparison of rectal mucosal cultures and fecal cultures in detecting salmonella infection in horses and cattle. Am J Vet Res 1985;46(3):697–8.

44. Burgess BA, Noyes NR, Bolte DS, et al. Rapid Salmonella detection in experimentally inoculated equine faecal and veterinary hospital environmental samples using commercially available lateral flow immunoassays. Equine Vet J 2015;47(1): 119–22.

45. Cohen ND, Neibergs HL, Wallis DE, et al. Genus-specific detection of salmonellae in equine feces by use of the polymerase chain reaction. Am J Vet Res 1994;55(8):1049–54.

46. Davies PR, Turkson PK, Funk JA, et al. Comparison of methods for isolating Salmonella bacteria from faeces of naturally infected pigs. J Appl Microbiol 2000; 89(1):169–77.

47. Cannon RM, Nicholls TJ. Relationship between sample weight, homogeneity, and sensitivity of fecal culture for Salmonella enterica. J Vet Diagn Invest 2002; 14(1):60–2.

48. Smith BP, Reina-Guerra M, Hardy AJ, et al. Equine salmonellosis: experimental production of four syndromes. Am J Vet Res 1979;40(8):1072–7.

49. Waltman WD, Mallinson ET. Isolation of Salmonella from poultry tissue and environmental samples: a nationwide survey. Avian Dis 1995;39:45–54.

50. Kuijpers A, Mooijman KA. EU Interlaboratory comparison study veterinary XV (2012): Detection of Salmonella in pig faeces. RIVM Rep 2013;330604028.

51. Ruple-Czerniak A, Bolte DS, Burgess BA, et al. Comparison of two sampling and culture systems for detection of Salmonella enterica in the environment of a large animal hospital. Equine Vet J 2014;46(4):499–502.

52. Burgess BA, Morley PS, Hyatt DR. Environmental surveillance for Salmonella enterica in a veterinary teaching hospital. J Am Vet Med Assoc 2004;225(9):1344–8.

53. Malorny B, Hoorfar J. Toward standardization of diagnostic PCR testing of fecal samples: lessons from the detection of salmonellae in pigs. J Clin Microbiol 2005;43(7):3033–7.

54. Cohen ND, Neibergs HL, McGruder ED, et al. Genus-specific detection of salmonellae using the polymerase chain reaction (PCR). J Vet Diagn Invest 1993;5(3): 368–71.

55. Kurowski PB, Traub-Dargatz JL, Morley PS, et al. Detection of Salmonella spp in fecal specimens by use of real-time polymerase chain reaction assay. Am J Vet Res 2002;63(9):1265–8.

56. Ward MP, Alinovi CA, Couetil LL, et al. Evaluation of a PCR to detect Salmonella in fecal samples of horses admitted to a veterinary teaching hospital. J Vet Diagn Invest 2005;17(2):118–23.

57. Ewart SL, Schott HC, 2nd, Robison RL, et al. Identification of sources of Salmonella organisms in a veterinary teaching hospital and evaluation of the effects of disinfectants on detection of Salmonella organisms on surface materials. J Am Vet Med Assoc 2001;218(7):1145–51.

58. Burgess BA, Weller CB, Pabilonia KL, et al. Detection of different serotypes of Salmonella enterica in experimentally inoculated equine fecal samples by commercially available rapid tests. *J Vet Intern Med* 2014;28(6):1853–9.
59. Bird CB, Miller RL, Miller BM. Reveal for Salmonella test system. J AOAC Int 1999; 82(3):625–33.
60. Castor ML, Wooley RE, Shotts EB, et al. Characteristics of Salmonella isolated from an outbreak of equine salmonellosis in a veterinary teaching hospital. *J Equine Vet Sci* 1989;9(5):236–41.

Potomac Horse Fever

Sandra D. Taylor, DVM, PhD

KEYWORDS

- Colitis • Diarrhea • Horse • Laminitis • Potomac • Sepsis

KEY POINTS

- *Neorickettsia risticii* and, less commonly, *N findlayensis*, are the causative agents of Potomac horse fever (PHF).
- Horses with PHF seem to have a higher risk of developing laminitis compared to horses with other causes of colitis.
- It is recommended that treatment of PHF with a tetracycline antibiotic is initiated immediately in euvolemic horses that have compatible clinical signs during the summer months in endemic regions.
- Although the currently available PHF vaccine might decrease incidence and severity of disease, it does not prevent infection.

INTRODUCTION

Potomac horse fever (PHF), also known as equine neorickettsiosis and equine monocytic ehrlichiosis, is a common cause of equine colitis in endemic areas. The disease was first reported near the Potomac River in Maryland in 1979 and since then, cases have been reported in North and South America.[1–5] Until recently, the only causative agent known to cause PHF was *Neorickettsia risticii* (formerly *Ehrlichia risticii*). However, a newly identified *Neorickettsia* spp., named *Neorickettsia findlayensis*, has been isolated from horses in Canada with PHF.[6,7] *Neorickettsia* spp. are intracellular, gram-negative bacteria of trematodes that parasitize aquatic insects (eg, caddisflies, mayflies, dragonflies, stoneflies, and damselflies) and snails.[8,9] Horses become infected upon ingestion of *Neorickettsia* spp.-infected trematodes within aquatic insects or within free-living trematodes.[10,11] Once inside the gastrointestinal tract, the bacteria are released from the trematode and invade colonic and cecal epithelial cells and tissue macrophages. Bacterial translocation into the blood leads to infection of monocytes. Given the intermediate hosts of *Neorickettsia* spp., disease is observed primarily in the summer and autumn months.[7,12,13]

Department of Veterinary Clinical Sciences, College of Veterinary Medicine, Purdue University, 625 Harrison Street, West Lafayette, IN 47907, USA
E-mail address: taylo248@purdue.edu

Vet Clin Equine 39 (2023) 37–45
https://doi.org/10.1016/j.cveq.2022.11.010
0749-0739/23/© 2022 Elsevier Inc. All rights reserved.

Clinical Presentation

The most commonly reported clinical signs in horses with PHF include diarrhea, fever, anorexia, lethargy, and colic.[7,12] One study found that 93% of horses diagnosed with PHF had diarrhea and/or fever.[7] Among horses with diarrhea from PHF, fecal consistency varies widely from watery, "pipe-stream" diarrhea (**Fig. 1**) to soft-formed feces. Milder presentations occur such that the degree of colitis does not overwhelm the colon's resorptive capacity; in these cases, inappetence and lethargy may be the predominant signs. Systemic inflammatory response syndrome (SIRS) might result from severe intestinal mucosal injury and bacterial translocation of normal intestinal flora into circulation.[14] Endotoxemia refers specifically to Gram-negative bacteria in the blood and is a common cause of SIRS in horses with colitis.[15] In horses with SIRS from PHF, other clinical signs such as tachycardia, tachypnea, toxic mucous membranes (**Fig. 2**), and laminitis might occur. Laminitis has been reported to occur in 22% to 42% of PHF cases.[7,12,16] Horses with PHF seem to have a higher risk of developing laminitis compared to horses with other causes of colitis.[12,16–18] The classic stance of a horse with bilateral front limb laminitis is shown in **Fig. 3**. Abortion as a result of acute PHF during pregnancy and subsequent vertical transmission has been reported and can occur months after clinical recovery of the mare.[19,20]

Neutropenia is a common initial finding in horses with PHF since neutrophils extravasate to the gastrointestinal tract during the innate immune response to infection.[12,21,22] Common biochemical abnormalities include hypocalcemia, hyponatremia, hypochloremia, and hypoproteinemia due to loss through the damaged colonic wall.[12,23] Indices of dehydration and hypovolemia from decreased fluid intake and diarrhea might be present, including increased hematocrit, red blood cells, L-lactate concentration, and pre-renal azotemia.[12]

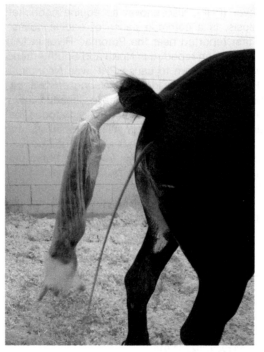

Fig. 1. "Pipe-stream" profuse, watery diarrhea in a horse with PHF.

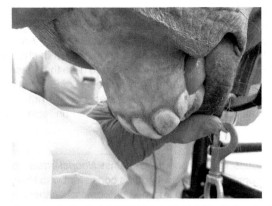

Fig. 2. Mucous membranes of a horse with PHF showing a "toxic line" adjacent to the incisors due to endotoxemia/SIRS.

Diagnostic Tests

The diagnostic test of choice for PHF is polymerase chain reaction (PCR) of blood and feces.[12] *N risticii* is likely to be detected by PCR in whole blood before and for a longer period of time compared with feces. Experimental infection with *N risticii* resulted in positive whole blood PCR from approximately 7–21 days post-infection, compared with fecal PCR positivity that was detected from approximately 11–16 days post-infection.[8,24] A real-time PCR test has recently been developed to specifically identify *N findlayensis*, although differentiating between *N risticii* and *N findlayensis* is likely clinically unnecessary with respect to treatment and outcome. Bacterial culture of *N risticii* or *N findlayensis* remains the reference standard of diagnosis, but delayed results coupled with the relatively high sensitivity and specificity of combined whole blood and fecal PCR testing often preclude its use in a clinical setting.[25] Serologic testing, including indirect fluorescent antibody testing and ELISA, is not recommended due to high variation in single and convalescent titers.[12,26]

The most common differential diagnoses for horses with PHF include colitis and/or typhlitis caused by *Salmonella* spp., *Clostridium perfringens* Types A and C, *Clostridioides difficile* and equine coronavirus. Ruling out disease caused by these infections might be necessary in horses with suspected PHF. Antemortem diagnosis of

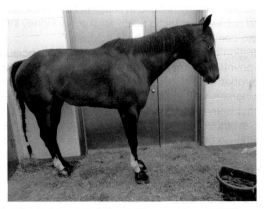

Fig. 3. A horse with bilateral front limb laminitis secondary to PHF.

Salmonella spp. infection can be made by fecal PCR and/or fecal culture. Typically, 3–5 serial fecal samples are required for PCR or culture, depending on the laboratory requirements, to account for intermittent fecal shedding.[27–29] Anaerobic fecal culture with subsequent PCR for toxin genes is the diagnostic test of choice for *C perfringens* and *C. difficile* infections, although it is important to note that these organisms can be found in the gastrointestinal tract of healthy horses.[30–32] Enzyme immunoassays that detect fecal toxin proteins have been developed but are not widely available.[30,33] Antemortem diagnosis of equine coronavirus is based on fecal PCR.[34]

Treatment and Supportive Care

Tetracycline antibiotics remain effective against *Neorickettsia* spp., and the use of oxytetracycline in horses with clinical findings consistent with PHF, even before definitive diagnosis, has been shown to improve outcomes.[12] Although the use of tetracyclines has been shown to prolong shedding of *Salmonella* spp. in experimentally infected ponies, it is recommended to treat horses with signs consistent with PHF in endemic areas during summer and autumn months to increase the likelihood for survival.[12,35]

Supportive care is a critical component of therapy in most of the horses with PHF. Fluid therapy in horses with gastrointestinal disease has been discussed in depth elsewhere.[36–39] Briefly, a fluid therapy plan should include three components: (1) replacing the fluid deficit; (2) providing maintenance fluids; and (3) replacing ongoing fluid losses (if applicable). The fluid deficit is calculated using the following formula:

Fluid deficit (L) = body weight (kg) x % dehydration

The percentage of dehydration is estimated based on skin turgor, eye position, corneal moisture, and mucous membrane moisture. The maintenance fluid rate for an adult horse is approximately 60 mL/kg/d and includes insensible fluid losses from respiration and sweating. Ongoing fluid losses can be due to diarrhea, polyuria, excessive salivation, and gastric reflux.

In addition to volume replacement, the goal of fluid therapy is to correct acid-base and electrolyte disturbances when applicable. Many horses with colitis will be dehydrated and hypovolemic with electrolyte loss (as described above) and metabolic acidosis.[18,40,41] In most of the cases, initial fluid resuscitation with isotonic crystalloids is sufficient. Fluid additives such as potassium chloride and/or calcium gluconate might be indicated once a resuscitation bolus has been administered. Sodium bicarbonate supplementation is rarely needed in cases of PHF since acidosis is largely due to hypovolemia and subsequent lactic acidosis; if acute kidney injury is present, uremic acids might also contribute to metabolic acidosis.[42]

Colloid administration can be beneficial in providing oncotic support. Horses with PHF are often hypovolemic and hypoalbuminemic, the latter of which is due to protein-losing enteropathy. Since albumin is the primary determinant of plasma oncotic pressure, horses with colitis often have a low colloid osmotic pressure (COP).[43,44] The most commonly used colloids in equine medicine are commercial equine plasma and synthetic colloids such as hydroxyethyl starches (HES). One study found that in healthy horses, plasma and HES increased COP to a similar, albeit modest, degree.[45] In a retrospective study of horses with enterocolitis, horses treated with plasma were more likely to survive than horses treated with HES (80% vs 47% survival; $P = .041$), after accounting for confounding variables.[46] This suggests that plasma might be superior to HES in the treatment of PHF, but prospective clinical trials are warranted. The benefit of plasma over HES includes the provision of albumin, coagulation factors, and immunoglobulins, whereas the benefits of HES over plasma include lower cost and higher oncotic pressure.[45,47]

Nonsteroidal anti-inflammatory drugs (NSAIDs; eg, flunixin meglumine) are important in addressing intestinal inflammation, SIRS, and laminitis. Is it important to restore hydration before administering NSAIDs to decrease the risk of NSAID-associated acute kidney injury.[48] Prophylactic anti-ulcer medication is recommended in anorexic or inappetence horses.[49] Polymyxin B is an antimicrobial drug that can be administered IV to bind circulating endotoxin,[50-55] but should be used with caution in hypovolemic horses given its potential nephrotoxic effects.[50]

Specific treatments for laminitis include NSAIDs, continuous digital cryotherapy, lidocaine as a continuous rate infusion, opioids, solar support, and in severe cases, coronary band grooving and foot casts.[16,56,57] Prophylactic continuous digital cryotherapy has been shown to reduce the risk of laminitis development in horses with colitis.[58] Laminitis treatment has been discussed in depth elsewhere.[56]

Prognosis

The survival rate for horses with PHF that is presented to a tertiary care facility is approximately 70%.[12,16,18] Horses with PHF that are treated with a tetracycline antibiotic are more likely to survive, and horses with clinicopathological findings consistent with hypovolemia, such as pre-renal azotemia and decreased serum electrolyte concentrations, are less likely to survive.[12] Laminitis as a risk factor for non-survival in horses with PHF is inconsistently reported and is likely a reflection of disease severity, prognosis for return to work, and financial constraints.[12,16,58] Severity of illness depends on several pathogen and host factors including *Neorickettsia* spp. strain, pathogenicity, and quantity ingested, as well as host immunocompetence, concurrent stress or illness, long-distance travel and pregnancy.[59,60]

Prevention

Four PHF vaccines containing a liquid suspension of inactivated *N risticii* have been licensed for use in the United States, with one vaccine currently available. It has been shown, however, that administering killed *N risticii* bacterin fails to mitigate clinical sings or reduce treatment costs.[61] Vaccine failure is due, at least in part, to various strains of *N risticii* expressing different major antigens.[59,60] Vaccine failure has been reported to be 82% to 89% and is associated with relatively low levels of vaccine-induced antibodies.[12,60] *N risticii* strains lack conserved immunogenic surface proteins that are able to elicit a broadly reactive adaptive immune response in affected horses.[60] A cross-protective vaccine will likely require multiple strains or conserved peptides.

Strategies to reduce exposure to intermediate hosts of *Neorickettsia* spp can be implemented to decrease the risk of PHF. Turning barn lights off at dusk can decrease exposure to freshwater flies, and preventing horses from drinking water from natural sources can decrease exposure to free-living flukes.

CLINICS CARE POINTS

- The most common clinical signs in horses with Potomac horse fever (PHF) are anorexia, fever, and diarrhea.
- Common clinicopathological abnormalities in horses with PHF include neutropenia, increased hematocrit, hypocalcemia, hyponatremia, hypochloremia, and hypoproteinemia.

- The diagnostic test of choice for PHF is polymerase chain reaction of both whole blood and feces.
- In addition to treatment with a tetracycline antibiotic, additional therapies for PHF might include intravenous fluid therapy, nonsteroidal anti-inflammatory drugs, digital cryotherapy, and anti-endotoxin therapy.

DISCLOSURE

The author has nothing to disclose.

REFERENCES

1. Dutra F, Schuch LF, Delucchi E, et al. Equine monocytic Ehrlichiosis (Potomac horse fever) in horses in Uruguay and southern Brazil. J Vet Diagn Invest 2001; 13:433–7.
2. Paulino PG, Almosny N, Oliveira R, et al. Detection of Neorickettsia risticii, the agent of Potomac horse fever, in horses from Rio de Janeiro, Brazil. Sci Rep 2020;10:7208.
3. Shapiro J, Thomson G. Potomac horse fever in eastern Ontario. Can Vet J 1995; 36:448.
4. Ehrich M, Perry BD, Troutt HF, et al. Acute diarrhea in horses of the Potomac River area: examination for clostridial toxins. J Am Vet Med Assoc 1984;185:433–5.
5. Knowles RC, Anderson CW, Shipley WD, et al. Acute equine diarrhea syndrome (AEDS): a preliminary report. Dallas, TX: American Association of Equine Practitioners; 1984. p. 353–7.
6. Teymournejad O, Lin M, Bekebrede H, et al. Isolation and Molecular Analysis of a Novel Neorickettsia Species That Causes Potomac Horse Fever. mBio 2020; 11(1):e03429–519.
7. Arroyo LG, Moore A, Bedford S, et al. Potomac horse fever in Ontario: Clinical, geographic, and diagnostic aspects. Can Vet J 2021;62:622–8.
8. Pusterla N, Madigan JE, Chae JS, et al. Helminthic transmission and isolation of Ehrlichia risticii, the causative agent of Potomac horse fever, by using trematode stages from freshwater stream snails. J Clin Microbiol 2000;38:1293–7.
9. Chae JS, Pusterla N, Johnson E, et al. Infection of aquatic insects with trematode metacercariae carrying Ehrlichia risticii, the cause of Potomac horse fever. J Med Entomol 2000;37:619–25.
10. Park BK, Kim MJ, Kim EH, et al. Identification of trematode cercariae carrying Neorickettsia risticii in freshwater stream snails. Ann N Y Acad Sci 2003;990: 239–47.
11. Madigan JE, Pusterla N, Johnson E, et al. Transmission of Ehrlichia risticii, the agent of Potomac horse fever, using naturally infected aquatic insects and helminth vectors: preliminary report. Equine Vet J 2000;32:275–9.
12. Bertin FR, Reising A, Slovis NM, et al. Clinical and clinicopathological factors associated with survival in 44 horses with equine neorickettsiosis (Potomac horse Fever). J Vet Intern Med 2013;27:1528–34.
13. Uzal FA, Arroyo LG, Navarro MA, et al. Bacterial and viral enterocolitis in horses: a review. J Vet Diagn Invest 2022;34:354–75.
14. Taylor S. A review of equine sepsis. Equine Vet Educ 2015;27:99–109.
15. Werners AH, Bull S, Fink-Gremmels J. Endotoxaemia: a review with implications for the horse. Equine Vet J 2005;37:371–83.

16. Luethy D, Feldman R, Stefanovski D, et al. Risk factors for laminitis and nonsurvival in acute colitis: Retrospective study of 85 hospitalized horses (2011-2019). J Vet Intern Med 2021;35:2019–25.

17. Manship AJ, Blikslager AT, Elfenbein JR. Disease features of equine coronavirus and enteric salmonellosis are similar in horses. J Vet Intern Med 2019;33:912–7.

18. Gomez DE, Leclere M, Arroyo LG, et al. Acute diarrhea in horses: A multicenter Canadian retrospective study (2015 to 2019). Can Vet J 2022;63:1033–42.

19. Long MT, Goetz TE, Kakoma I, et al. Evaluation of fetal infection and abortion in pregnant ponies experimentally infected with Ehrlichia risticii. Am J Vet Res 1995; 56:1307–16.

20. Coffman EA, Abd-Eldaim M, Craig LE. Abortion in a horse following Neorickettsia risticii infection. J Vet Diagn Invest 2008;20:827–30.

21. Ziemer EL, Whitlock RH, Palmer JE, et al. Clinical and hematologic variables in ponies with experimentally induced equine ehrlichial colitis (Potomac horse fever). Am J Vet Res 1987;48:63–7.

22. Cordes DO, Perry BD, Rikihisa Y, et al. Enterocolitis caused by Ehrlichia sp. in the horse (Potomac horse fever). Vet Pathol 1986;23:471–7.

23. Rikihisa Y, Johnson GC, Wang YZ, et al. Loss of absorptive capacity for sodium and chloride in the colon causes diarrhoea in Potomac horse fever. Res Vet Sci 1992;52:353–62.

24. Biswas B, Vemulapalli R, Dutta SK. Detection of Ehrlichia risticii from feces of infected horses by immunomagnetic separation and PCR. J Clin Microbiol 1994;32: 2147–51.

25. Mott J, Rikihisa Y, Zhang Y, et al. Comparison of PCR and culture to the indirect fluorescent-antibody test for diagnosis of Potomac horse fever. J Clin Microbiol 1997;35:2215–9.

26. Madigan JE, Rikihisa Y, Palmer JE, et al. Evidence for a high rate of false-positive results with the indirect fluorescent antibody test for Ehrlichia risticii antibody in horses. J Am Vet Med Assoc 1995;207:1448–53.

27. Kurowski PB, Traub-Dargatz JL, Morley PS, et al. Detection of Salmonella spp in fecal specimens by use of real-time polymerase chain reaction assay. Am J Vet Res 2002;63:1265–8.

28. Cohen ND, Martin LJ, Simpson RB, et al. Comparison of polymerase chain reaction and microbiological culture for detection of salmonellae in equine feces and environmental samples. Am J Vet Res 1996;57:780–6.

29. Alinovi CA, Ward MP, Couetil LL, et al. Risk factors for fecal shedding of Salmonella from horses in a veterinary teaching hospital. Prev Vet Med 2003;60:307–17.

30. Silva RO, Ribeiro MG, Palhares MS, et al. Detection of A/B toxin and isolation of clostridium difficile and clostridium perfringens from foals. Equine Vet J 2013;45: 671–5.

31. Wierup M, DiPietro JA. Bacteriologic examination of equine fecal flora as a diagnostic tool for equine intestinal clostridiosis. Am J Vet Res 1981;42:2167–9.

32. Schoster A, Kunz T, Lauper M, et al. Prevalence of Clostridium difficile and Clostridium perfringens in Swiss horses with and without gastrointestinal disease and microbiota composition in relation to Clostridium difficile shedding. Vet Microbiol 2019;239:108433.

33. Ramos CP, Lopes EO, Oliveira Junior CA, et al. Immunochromatographic test and ELISA for the detection of glutamate dehydrogenase (GDH) and A/B toxins as an alternative for the diagnosis of Clostridioides (Clostridium) difficile-associated diarrhea in foals and neonatal piglets. Braz J Microbiol 2020;51:1459–62.

34. Pusterla N, Mapes S, Wademan C, et al. Emerging outbreaks associated with equine coronavirus in adult horses. Vet Microbiol 2013;162:228–31.

35. Owen RA, Fullerton J, Barnum DA. Effects of transportation, surgery, and anti-biotic therapy in ponies infected with Salmonella. Am J Vet Res 1983;44:46–50.

36. Shaw SD, Stampfli H. Diagnosis and treatment of undifferentiated and infectious acute diarrhea in the adult horse. Vet Clin North Am Equine Pract 2018;34:39–53.

37. Seahorn JL, Seahorn TL. Fluid therapy in horses with gastrointestinal disease. Vet Clin North Am Equine Pract 2003;19:665–79.

38. Freeman DE. Fluid therapy in horses: how much is too much? Vet Rec 2021;188: 103–5.

39. Crabtree NE, Epstein KL. Current concepts in fluid therapy in horses. Front Vet Sci 2021;8:648774.

40. Ecke P, Hodgson DR, Rose RJ. Induced diarrhoea in horses. part 1: fluid and electrolyte balance. Vet J 1998;155:149–59.

41. Stewart MC, Hodgson JL, Kim H, et al. Acute febrile diarrhoea in horses: 86 cases (1986-1991). Aust Vet J 1995;72:41–4.

42. Gomez DE, Arroyo LG, Stampfli HR, et al. Physicochemical interpretation of acid-base abnormalities in 54 adult horses with acute severe colitis and diarrhea. J Vet Intern Med 2013;27:548–53.

43. Bellezzo F, Kuhnmuench T, Hackett ES. The effect of colloid formulation on colloid osmotic pressure in horses with naturally occurring gastrointestinal disease. BMC Vet Res 2014;10(Suppl 1):S8.

44. Arroyo LG, Sears W, Gomez DE. Plasma transfusions in horses with typhlocolitis/colitis. Can Vet J 2019;60:193–6.

45. McKenzie EC, Esser MM, McNitt SE, et al. Effect of infusion of equine plasma or 6% hydroxyethyl starch (600/0.75) solution on plasma colloid osmotic pressure in healthy horses. Am J Vet Res 2016;77:708–14.

46. Kopper JJ, Kogan CJ, Cook VL, et al. Outcome of horses with enterocolitis receiving oncotic fluid support with either plasma or hetastarch. Can Vet J 2019;60:1207–12.

47. van Galen G, Hallowell G. Hydroxyethyl starches in equine medicine. J Vet Emerg Crit Care (San Antonio) 2019;29:349–59.

48. Gunson DE, Soma LR. Renal papillary necrosis in horses after phenylbutazone and water deprivation. Vet Pathol 1983;20:603–10.

49. Bishop RC, Kemper AM, Wilkins PA, et al. Effect of omeprazole and sucralfate on gastrointestinal injury in a fasting/NSAID model. Equine Vet J 2021. https://doi.org/10.1111/evj.13534.

50. MacKay RJ, Clark CK, Logdberg L, et al. Effect of a conjugate of polymyxin B-dextran 70 in horses with experimentally induced endotoxemia. Am J Vet Res 1999;60:68–75.

51. Wong DM, Sponseller BA, Alcott CJ, et al. Effects of intravenous administration of polymyxin B in neonatal foals with experimental endotoxemia. J Am Vet Med As-soc 2013;243:874–81.

52. Barton MH, Parviainen A, Norton N. Polymyxin B protects horses against induced endotoxaemia in vivo. Equine Vet J 2004;36:397–401.

53. Morresey PR, Mackay RJ. Endotoxin-neutralizing activity of polymyxin B in blood after IV administration in horses. Am J Vet Res 2006;67:642–7.

54. Durando MM, Mackay RJ, Linda S, et al. Effects of polymyxin-B and salmonella-typhimurium antiserum on horses given endotoxin intravenously. Am J Vet Res 1994;55:921–7.

55. Parviainen AK, Barton MH, Norton NN. Evaluation of polymyxin B in an ex vivo model of endotoxemia in horses. Am J Vet Res 2001;62(1):72–6.
56. Leise BS, Fugler LA. Laminitis Updates: Sepsis/Systemic Inflammatory Response Syndrome-Associated Laminitis. Vet Clin North Am Equine Pract 2021;37:639–56.
57. Stokes SM, Belknap JK, Engiles JB, et al. Continuous digital hypothermia prevents lamellar failure in the euglycaemic hyperinsulinaemic clamp model of equine laminitis. Equine Vet J 2019;51:658–64.
58. Kullmann A, Holcombe SJ, Hurcombe SD, et al. Prophylactic digital cryotherapy is associated with decreased incidence of laminitis in horses diagnosed with colitis. Equine Vet J 2014;46:554–9.
59. Biswas B, Vemulapalli R, Dutta SK. Molecular basis for antigenic variation of a protective strain-specific antigen of Ehrlichia risticii. Infect Immun 1998;66:3682–8.
60. Dutta SK, Vemulapalli R, Biswas B. Association of deficiency in antibody response to vaccine and heterogeneity of Ehrlichia risticii strains with Potomac horse fever vaccine failure in horses. J Clin Microbiol 1998;36:506–12.
61. Atwill ER, Mohammed HO. Benefit-cost analysis of vaccination of horses as a strategy to control equine monocytic ehrlichiosis. J Am Vet Med Assoc 1996;208:1295–9.

Equine Rotaviral Diarrhea

Jamie J. Kopper, DVM, PhD, DACVIM-LAIM, DACVECC-LA

KEYWORDS

- Diarrhea • Foal • Vaccination

KEY POINTS

- Diarrhea due to equine rotavirus (ERV) is one of the most common causes of infectious diarrhea in foals.
- Diarrhea due to ERV is because of several mechanisms including malabsorption, temporary lactose intolerance, and activation of the enteric nervous system.
- Prevention relies on biosecurity and vaccination of pregnant mares followed by adequate ingestion of colostrum.

INTRODUCTION

Equine rotavirus (ERV) is endemic to horse populations and the most prevalent viral enteric pathogen in foals.[1] ERV belongs to the family Reoviridae, subfamily Sedoreovirinae and genus *Rotavirus*.[2] The virus was named for its wheel-like or icosahedral-shaped virions (Latin for wheel being "rota") that can be observed via electron microscopy.[3]

Rotaviruses are classified into groups A–H by the intermediate capsid protein VP6; however, until recently, only group A rotaviruses (ERVA) have been detected in horses.[4,5] In 2021, evidence for emergence of a group B (ERVB), ruminant origin rotavirus causing severe watery to hemorrhagic diarrhea was found in central Kentucky. Emergence of the ruminant-like group B rotavirus outbreak was reported from 22 farms in neonatal foals 2 to 7 days of age, a naïve population for this emergent virus.[6]

ERVs are nonenveloped viruses that contain 11 double-stranded RNA segments within their genome[7] with 2 outer capsid proteins referred to as VP4 and VP7. These capsid proteins elicit neutralizing antibodies and are used to classify ERVs into glycoprotein (G) and protease-sensitive (P) genotypes.[7] Epidemiologically, to date, most ERVAs are those classified as G3P[12] and G14P[12].[8] The recently detected ERVB virus was provisionally designated RVB/Horse-wt/USA/KY/1518/2021.[6]

Iowa State University, College of Veterinary Medicine, 1809 Christensen Drive, Ames Iowa 50010, USA
E-mail address: jkopper@iastate.edu

Vet Clin Equine 39 (2023) 47–54
https://doi.org/10.1016/j.cveq.2022.11.003
0749-0739/23/© 2022 Elsevier Inc. All rights reserved.

EPIDEMIOLOGY

ERV has been cited as the most frequently detected pathogen in foals with diarrhea,[4,9–11] is highly prevalent, and is considered endemic in most, if not all, horse populations worldwide. Diarrheal disease due to ERV has a seasonal association with most cases reported during spring and early summer, corresponding with foaling seasons.[12,13] Although ERV has been identified in the fecal material of apparently healthy foals,[11] it was uncommon, and those with ERV were significantly more likely to have concurrent diarrhea.

ERV is transmitted by fecal-oral route or by ingestion of contaminated fomites. Although intestinal disease due to rotavirus affects many species, including humans, cross-species transmission rarely occurs. Adult horses have not been reported to show clinical signs of disease; however, a small percentage of adults have evidence of shedding ERV in their manure (1.5%–3.4% of adult enteric disease panels more than a 4-year period),[14,15] thus serving as a potential source of infection to foals. Additionally, most adult horses have anti-ERV antibodies,[16,17] indicating exposure and potential subclinical infection. A minimum infective dose of ERV has not been established for foals. Research in piglets, however, has indicated that in piglets an inoculating dose as low as 90 virions can result in intestinal disease,[18] which is in stark contrast to the large amount of virions (10^{10}/g) in 1 g of pig feces.[18]

The potential role for ERV in enteric coinfections and disease severity in foals with diarrhea warrants further consideration. In one study, more than 50% of the foals with diarrhea were coinfected with another virus or parasite.[11] This is in contrast to adult horses, which are typically clinically unaffected by ERV, and a significant association with other enteric pathogens was not noted.[14] Similarly to foals, the potential role for ERV in coinfections of young people and animals has been noted in other species.[19,20] Interestingly, most research regarding coinfections with ERV have identified associations with other viral or parasitic pathogens, rather than bacterial pathogens. Currently, whether coinfections with ERV increase severity and/or length of disease and/or predispose patients to infection with other pathogens (or vice versa) is not well documented at this time.

PATHOGENESIS

Intestinal disease due to ERV infection is multifactorial—several of the mechanisms are outlined in later discussion. On ingestion, ERV infect differentiated enterocytes located within the mid to upper villi of the small intestine (duodenum, jejunum, and ileum) but leave the undifferentiated crypt cells unscathed.[21] After entering the enterocyte via Ca^{++}-dependent endocytosis, ERV replicates, and the enterocytes lyse on the release of virions resulting in cell death.[22] Loss of the infected enterocytes results in epithelial desquamation and shortening of the villi leading to decreased absorptive capacity and malabsorptive diarrhea.[23] Additionally, ERV infection negatively affects glucose absorption by 2 mechanisms. First, in addition to impairing Na + -glucose transport through inhibition of the sodium/glucose cotransporter 1 protein,[24] it also disrupts the mid to upper villi resulting in the destruction of the intestinal disaccharidases (sucrase, maltase, lactase) located within the brush-border membrane.[25] In pigs, rotaviral infection has been shown to notably reduce jejunal lactase activity.[26] This, effectively, results in temporary lactose intolerance of affected foals that are consuming an almost entirely milk-based diet, resulting in osmotic diarrhea. Furthermore, ERV likely activates the enteric nervous system (ENS) further contributing to the development of diarrhea. In a murine model of rotaviral diarrhea, the rotavirus-induced fluid secretory responses were decreased by greater than 60% when enteral neural blockers were coadministered.[27]

The effect of rotaviral infections on mucosal permeability has also been assessed in piglets.[26] Here, investigators found that while rotavirus infection did not have a significant effect on transepithelial resistance, intestinal permeability was increased as assessed by macromolecule flux and decreased cell membrane localization of occludin, a major tight junction protein.[26] Together, these results raise concern for associated loss of intestinal barrier integrity, which could predispose patients to translocation of intestinal bacteria and toxins further exacerbating disease.

Histologically, in addition to villus blunting, reported changes to the small intestinal epithelium include edema, mononuclear cell infiltrates, vacuolation, and the presence of viral particles within the cytoplasm.[16] Of note, due to the multifactorial mechanisms contributing to diarrhea, histologic lesions do not always correlate with severity of the diarrhea.[1]

CLINICAL DISEASE

Affected foals are between 2 and 253 days of age with a median age of 77 to 81 days at onset of clinical signs.[10,28] In general, ERV infection results in high morbidity but overall low mortality with 94% of affected foals surviving to discharge from a referral hospital in one study.[28] Clinically, foals usually present for decreased nursing behavior, lethargy, diarrhea, and may have pyrexia.[1] Affected foals less than 2 weeks of age have increased risk of worse disease severity and death,[11] with death most commonly occurring due to severe dehydration secondary to diarrhea. Affected foals may shed ERV 1 to 12 days before notable clinical signs (Bailey and colleagues 2013), however, and shedding may continue after the resolution of diarrhea.[29]

DIAGNOSTICS

Historically, a diagnosis of ERV relied on identifying ERV in fecal samples by electron microscopy and the gold standard for diagnosis of viral infections remains virus isolation and culture. That being said, these techniques are both costly and require significant expertise, thus may not be time sensitive. Given the importance of establishing a timely diagnosis, particularly for institution of appropriate biosecurity measures, the use of molecular-based technology such as real-time PCR and stall-side tests such as enzyme-linked immunosorbent assays (ELISAs), latex agglutination, and immunochromatographic assays are most commonly used. Many of the ELISA-based tests rely on the detection of antibodies to VP6, which is highly conserved across rotaviruses affecting multiple species. Considering this, several commercial human rotavirus detection kits have been assessed for diagnostic accuracy in foals with rotaviral diarrhea.[28,30] Human rotavirus detection kits have variable sensitivity and diagnostic accuracy in the horse[28,30] but some likely have value in situations where preliminary information will aide with rapid implementation of appropriate biosecurity protocols. As with other enteric pathogens (ie, *Salmonella* and Equine Coronavirus) intermittent shedding is possible,[5] particularly depending on when sampling is occurring in the stage of disease. Negative results should be interpreted in light of the clinical picture, diagnostic evaluation and reinterrogated if indicated.

Clinical signs associated with ERV infection do not distinguish affected foals from those afflicted by other infectious and noninfectious cases of diarrhea. Generally speaking, compared with foals affected by other infectious causes of diarrhea, foals with ERV have higher lymphocyte counts, decreased neutrophil toxicity and lower sepsis scores.[28] In another study evaluating serum amyloid A (SAA) as an aide in management of infectious disease in foals, they found that foals affected with ERV did not have a consistent inflammatory (SAA, fibrinogen, total leukocyte, neutrophil) response.[31]

TREATMENT

Disease due to ERV infection of foals is self-limiting, thus treatment is supportive and prophylactic in nature. Due to diarrhea, severely affected foals commonly need fluid therapy to both support hydration and manage any concurrent electrolyte derangements (ie, hyponatremia, metabolic acidosis, and so forth). The potential effects of rotaviral infections on intestinal permeability (ie, causes loss of intestinal barrier function and increases in permeability) may justify the use of broad-spectrum antimicrobials, in some cases, as prophylaxis for (or treatment of) secondary infection due to translocation of intestinal bacteria. However, the use of antimicrobials should be considered on a case-by-case basis in light of the individual foal's clinical signs and laboratory data. Depending on the age of the foal, assessment for failure of passive transfer (or immunoglobulin consumption) is warranted and treatment with plasma from immunized donors as needed.

Given the development and contribution of lactose intolerance to diarrhea and signs of colic in some ERV-infected foals, restricted nursing, short periods of intestinal rest and/or administration of supplemental lactase (120 U/kg PO q3-8 hours or before/with meal feeding) may decrease osmotic diarrhea fluid losses and signs of colic associated with the consumption of a milk-based diet in the face of temporary lactose intolerance. When instituting intestinal rest, use of partial or total parental nutrition should be considered. Provision of nutrition remains important for several reasons in foals. First, maintaining a positive or at least neutral energy balance is important for adequate immune function and tissue healing in critical illness. Second, the role of malnutrition in the course of infection with rotavirus has been a topic of interest in human children with rotavirus and piglet models of rotavirus infection. Malnourishment has been associated with prolonged rotavirus infection in piglets[32]; however, in a separate study, it did not have additive effects on intestinal barrier function in a piglet model.[26]

A relationship between ERV and gastroduodenal ulcers has been suggested,[33,34] and the use of proton pump inhibitors (PPIs) or histamine-type 2 (H2) antagonists and/or sucralfate has been promoted. However, the prophylactic use of PPIs or H2 antagonists remains an area of controversy given the association between use of PPIs or H2 antagonists and the development of undifferentiated diarrhea in hospitalized foals.[35]

PREVENTION

Other than good farm management and biosecurity practices, maternal vaccination remains the most widely used mechanism for the prevention of serious disease associated with ERV infection. With ERV infections occurring in foals as young as 2 days of age, and many affected foals being less than 1 month of age, direct vaccination of the foal is unlikely to be effective given their immature immune systems.[36] Worldwide, there are 3 inactivated vaccines (2 monovalent and 1 trivalent) licensed for use in pregnant mares to aide in providing passive transfer of antibodies to foals against ERV. Absent from the vaccination armamentarium is an ERVB vaccine addressing the newly identified virus. All 3 products currently available increase the presence of circulating anti-ERV antibodies in mares and foals.[37–39] A study evaluating the effects of an inactivated ERV vaccine in healthy prepartum broodmares found that when 3 vaccinations were delivered, 1 month apart, starting 4 months before parturition, the amount of ERV-specific IgG was increased at all time points (at parturition, 1, 7, 17, and

28 days postpartum) in mammary secretions and in foal serum (days 1, 7, and 28 postpartum) compared with mammary secretions and foals of unvaccinated mares. In these same mares and foals, there was no evidence of ERV-specific IgA in mammary secretions or foal serum at any time points. However, field studies have found mixed results in terms of efficacy in preventing ERV diarrhea in foals. In one study, there was no significant decrease in the incidence of ERV diarrhea in vaccinated versus unvaccinated foals,[39] whereas others found that foals of vaccinated mares had fewer clinical signs attributed to ERV diarrhea and fewer days of diarrhea.[37,38] These results may be further compounded by the reliance of adequate ingestion and absorption of appropriate quality colostrum by the foal to acquire ERV-specific IgG. Thus, the assessment of foals for failure of passive transfer and treatment with plasma transfusions from appropriately vaccinated donor herds may be a valuable part of the prevention plan. Together, studies indicate that although complete prevention of ERV in foals born to mares vaccinated for ERV is unlikely, vaccination may result in fewer days of diarrhea and decreased clinical signs associated with the disease.

Disinfection and containment are important components of ERV prevention and management as infected foals secrete large amounts of diarrhea (10^{10} virions/g of feces) and likely require a relatively small number of viral particles (<100) to cause disease. Although there is limited data regarding stability of ERV in the environment, bovine rotavirus is stable for 9 months in feces.[40] As a nonenveloped virus, ERA is more resistant to hostile environmental conditions and disinfectants that enveloped equine viruses, such as equine herpes viruses and influenza virus.

For hand hygiene of personnel working with affected foals, chlorohexidine solutions alone are ineffective. In the presence of organic material, however, several options have demonstrated efficacy, including 10% providone iodine, 70% ethanol or isopropanol, and 1.5% chlorhexidine/15% cetrimide/70% ethanol.[41,42] However, the shear volume of organic material in equine facilities makes environmental decontamination challenging because the efficacy of most disinfectants is negatively influenced by the presence of notable organic debris. In general, amphoteric soaps and quaternary ammonium compounds are ineffective against ERV.[43] Although virucidal effects of chlorine-based and iodine-based infectants are negatively affected by the presence of organic material, they are not notably decreased by temperature,[43] unlike glutaraldehyde, where the efficacy is negative influenced by low temperatures[43] facing many practitioners and farms. When disinfecting barns and personnel, as much organic material should be removed as possible before the application of disinfectants, and foot mats should be frequently changed to prevent the accumulation of organic debris thus decreasing efficacy.

SUMMARY

In summary, infection with ERV causes diarrhea in foals 2 days to 252 days of age (average 77–88 days) that generally has low mortality rates with appropriate supportive care. Diarrhea in foals with ERV is because of several mechanisms including loss of absorptive surfaces and capacity, development of temporary lactose intolerance, and activation of the ENS. Infection with ERV is self-limiting, meaning that the treatment is supportive in nature and often involves correction of dehydration and electrolyte imbalances due to large volumes of diarrhea. Prevention is aimed at delivery of ERV-specific IgG in colostrum by vaccinating pregnant mares and biosecurity practices, although neither fully prevents the development of diarrhea due to ERV. Detection and characterization of ERVB in foals indicate the need for an expanded vaccine repertoire and vigilance for zoonotic potential in other species, including humans.

CLINICS CARE POINTS

- Treatment of rotaviral diarrhea is supportive in nature. Based on severity of illness, attention should be paid to hydration, electrolyte and acid-base status.
- Rotaviral diarrhea should be considered in foals with diarrhea between 2 and 252 days of age (average 77-88).
- Equine rotavirus is easily transmittable between foals, thus quarnatine and biosecurity is important in limiting spread of on-farm infection.

DISCLOSURE

The author does not have any relevant commercial or financial conflicts of interest to claim. There are no funding sources to disclose.

REFERENCES

1. Bailey K, Gilkerson J, Browning G. Equine rotaviruses – current understanding and continued challenges. Vet Microbiol 2013;167:135–44.
2. Carstens E. Ratification vote on taxonomic proposals to the International Committee on Taxonomy of Viruses (2009). Arch Virol 2010;155:133–46.
3. Flewett T, Bryden A, Davies H, et al. Relation between viruses from acute gastroenteritis of children and new born calves. Lancet 1974;2:61–3.
4. Browning G, Chalmers R, Snodgrass D, et al. The prevalence of enteric pathogens in diarrheic thoroughbred foals in Britain and Ireland. Equine Vet J 1991; 23:405–9.
5. Magdesian K, Dwyer R, Arguedas M. Viral Diarrhea. In: Sellon D, Long M, editors. Equine infectious diseases. Saint Louis: WB Sanders; 2014. p. 198–201.
6. Uprety T, Sreenviasan CC, Hause BM, et al. Identification of a ruminant origin group B rotavirus associated with diarrhea outbreaks in foals. Viruses 2021; 13(7):1330.
7. Estes M, Greenberg H. Rotaviruses. In: Knipe D, Howel P, editors. Fields virology. 6th Edition. Philadelphia: Lippincott Williams & Wilkins; 2013. p. 1347–401.
8. Papp H, Matthijnssesn J, Martella V, et al. Global distribution of group A rotavirus strains in horses: a systemic review. Vaccine 2013;31:5627–33.
9. Netherwood T, Wood J, Townsend H, et al. Foal diarrhoea between 1991 and 1994 in the United Kingdom associated with Clostridium perfringens, rotavirus, Strongyloides westeri and Cryptosporidium spp. Epidemiol Infect 1996;117:375–83.
10. Dwyer R, Powell D, Roberts W, et al. A study of the etiology and control of infectious diarrhea among foals in central Kentucky. Proc Am Assoc Equine Pract 1990;36:337–55.
11. Slovis N, Elam J, Strada M, et al. Infectious agents associated with diarrhoea in neonatal foals in central Kentucky: A comprehensive molecular study. Equine Vet J 2014;46:311–6.
12. Collins P, Cullinane A, Martella V, et al. molecular characterization of equine rotavirus in Ireland. J Clin Microbiol 2008;46:3346–54.
13. Ntafis V, Fragkadaki E, Xylouri E, et al. Rotavirus-associated diarrhoea in foals in Greece. Vet Micribiol 2010;144:461–5.
14. Kopper J, Willette J, Kogan C, et al. Detection of pathogens in blood or feces of adult horses with enteric disease and association with outcome of colitis. J Vet Intern Med 2021;35:2465–72.

15. Willete J, Kopper J, Kogan C, et al. Effect of season and geographic location in the United States on detection of potential enteric pathogens of toxin genes in horses ≥ 6 mo-old. J Vet Diagn Invest 2021;32:407–11.
16. Conner M, Darlington R. Rotavirus infection in foals. Am J Vet Res 1980;41: 1699–703.
17. Goto H, Tsunemitsu H, Horitomo M, et al. A sero-epidemiological study on rotavirus infection in horses. Bull Equine Res Inst 1981;18:129–35.
18. Payment P, Morin E. Minimal infective dose of the OSU strain of porcine rotavirus. Arch Virol 1990;112:277–82.
19. Delling C, Daughshchies A. Literature review: coinfection in young ruminant livestock - Cryptosporidium spp and its companions. Pathogens 2022;11(1):103.
20. Koh H, Baek J, Shin J, et al. Coinfection of viral agents in Korean children with acute watery diarrhea. J Korean Med Sci 2008;23:937–40.
21. Ciarlet M, Estes M. Interactions between rotavirus and gastrointestinal cells. Curr Opin Microbiol 2001;4:435–41.
22. Ruiz M, Cohen J, Michelangeli F. Role of Ca2+ in the replication and pathogenesis of rotavirus and other viral infections. Cell Calcium 2000;28:137–49.
23. Woode G, Crouch C. Naturally occurring and experimentally induced rotaviral infections of domestic and laboratory animals. J Am Vet Med Assoc 1978;173: 522–6.
24. Halaihel N, Lieven V, Alvarado F, et al. Rotavrius infection impairs intestinal brush-border membrane Na(+)-solute cotransport activities in young rabbits. Am J Physiol Gastrointest Liver Physiol 2000;279:G587–96.
25. Collins J, Starkley W, Wallis T, et al. Intestinal enzyme profiles in normal and rotavirus-infected mice. J Pediatr Gastroenterol Nutr 1988;7:264–72.
26. Jacobi S, Moeser A, Blikslager A, et al. Acute effects of rotavirus and malnutrition on intestinal barrier function in neonatal piglets. World J Gastroenterol 2013;19: 5094–102.
27. Lundgren A, Peregrin A, Persson K, et al. Role of the enteric nervous system in the fluid and electrolyte secretion of rotavirus diarrhea. Science 2000;287:491–5.
28. Frederick J, Giguere S, Sanchez L. Infectious agents detected in the feces of diarrheic foals: a retrospective study of 233 cases (2003-2008). J Vet Intern Med 2009;23:1254–60.
29. Ciarlet M, Conner E, et al. Antigenic and molecular analyses reveal that the equine rotavirus strain H-1 is closely related to porcie but not equine, rotaviruses: interspecies transmission from pigs to horses? Virus Genes 2001;22:5–20.
30. Mino S, Kern A, Barrandeguy M, et al. Comparison of two commercial kits and an in house ELISA for the detection of equine rotavirus in foal feces. J Virol Methods 2015;222:1–10.
31. Hulten C, Demmers S. Serum amyloid A (SAA) as an aid in the management of infectious disease in the foal: comparison with total leucocyte count, neutrophil count and fibrinogen. Equine Vet J 2002;34:693–8.
32. Zijlstra R, Donoval S, Olde J, et al. Protein-energy malnutrition delays small-intestinal recovery in neonatal pigs infected with rotavirus. J Nutr 1997;127: 1118–27.
33. Murray MJ, Murray CM, Sweeney HJ, et al. Prevalence of gastric lesions in foals without signs of gastric disease: an endoscopic survey. Equine Vet J 1990; 22:6–8.
34. Taharaguchi S, Okai K, Orita Y, et al. Association between diarrhea and gastric or duodenal lesions in foals in Hidaka, Japan. J Jpn Vet Med Assoc 2007;60: 569–72.

35. Furr M, Cohen N, Axon J, et al. Treatment with histamine-type 2 receptor antagonists and omeprazole increase the risk of diarrhoea in neonatal foals treated in intensive care units. Equine Vet J 2012;44:80–6.
36. Nemoto J, Matsumara T. Equine rotavirus infection. J Equine Sci 2021;32:1–9.
37. Barrandeguy M, Parreno V, Lagos Marmol M, et al. Prevention of rotavirus diarrhoea in foals by parenteral vaccination of the mares: field trial. Dev Biol Stand 1998;92:253–7.
38. Imagawa H, Kato T, Tsunemitsu H, et al. Field study of inactivated equine rotavirus vaccine. J Equine Sci 2005;16:35–44.
39. Powell D, Dwyer R, Traub-Dargatz J, et al. Field study of the safety, immunogenicity and efficacy of an inactivated equine rotavirus. J Am Vet Med Assoc 1997;211:193–8.
40. Woode G. Epizootiology of bovine rotavirus infection. Vet Rec 1978;103:44–6.
41. Sattar S, Raphael R, Lochnan H, et al. Rotavirus inactivation by chemical disinfectants and antiseptics used in hospitals. Can J Microbiol 1983;29:1464–9.
42. Springthrope V, Grenier J, Lloydevans N, et al. Chemical disinfection of human rotaviruses – efficacy of commercially available products in suspension tests. J Hyg 1983;97:139–61.
43. Nemoto N, Bannai H, Tsujinmura K, et al. Virucidal effect of commercially available disinfectants of equine group A rotavirus. J Vet Med Sci 2014;76:1061–3.

Equine Coronaviruses

Nicola Pusterla, DVM, PhD

KEYWORDS

- Equine coronavirus (ECoV)
- Severe acute respiratory syndrome coronavirus-2 (SARS-CoV-2) • Epidemiology
- Pathogenesis • Clinical signs • Diagnosis • Treatment and prevention

KEY POINTS

- Equids are susceptible to severe acute respiratory syndrome coronavirus-2 (SARS-CoV-2) based on the high homology to the ACE-2 receptor; however, only silent infection has been documented now.
- Equine coronavirus (ECoV) infection in adult equids is often characterized by unspecific clinical signs such as fever, lethargy, and anorexia, whereas changes in fecal character and colic are infrequently observed in infected animals.
- A diagnosis of ECoV should be considered when multiple adult horses are affected by fever, lethargy, anorexia with or without gastrointestinal signs and hematological changes (leukopenia due to neutropenia and/or lymphopenia) are consistent with an underlying viral disease. A laboratory diagnosis of ECoV is supported by the molecular detection of ECoV in feces.
- ECoV infection is often self-limiting requiring at best supportive treatment with non-steroidal antiinflammatory drugs and polyionic fluids and antimicrobials if endotoxemia/septicemia is suspected.
- The prevention of ECoV infection should focus on the implementation of routine management practices aimed at reducing the likelihood of introducing and disseminating ECoV at any horse-based premise as well as the timely isolation of horses with suspected ECoV infection.

SEVERE ACUTE RESPIRATORY SYNDROME CORONAVIRUS 2

Although successful experimental transmission of severe acute respiratory syndrome coronavirus-2 (SARS-CoV-2) has been documented in a variety of domestic and laboratory animal species, including dogs, cats, ferrets, pigs, New Zealand white rabbits, mice, and Syrian hamsters,[1-5] suspected natural transmission through the spillover from infected humans to domestic animals has only been reported in dogs and cats.[6-11] Susceptibility and exposure to SARS-CoV-2 are the 2 main prerequisites for any domestic animal to develop clinical or subclinical infection.[12] Less research

Department of Medicine and Epidemiology, School of Veterinary Medicine, University of California, One Shields Avenue, Davis, CA 95616, USA
E-mail address: npusterla@ucdavis.edu

Vet Clin Equine 39 (2023) 55–71
https://doi.org/10.1016/j.cveq.2022.11.008
0749-0739/23/© 2022 Elsevier Inc. All rights reserved.
vetequine.theclinics.com

has been focusing on characterizing the role of equids in the COVID-19 pandemic. Susceptibility of equids (horses and donkeys) has been established by comparative analysis of ACE-2 protein sequences, and the data showed that equids have low affinity to bind.[13] A recent functional and genetic study determined that viral receptor ACE-2 orthologs from 44 different species, including horses, were able to bind SARS-CoV-2 spike protein, therefore supporting viral entry.[14]

Experimental intranasal infection with an ancestral SARS-CoV-2 strain (virus strain 2019-nCoV/USA-WA1/2020) in a single horse has been reported in the literature (**Table 1**).[15] The attempt to experimentally infect the single horse failed, which is not surprising, considering that experimental infections of equids using the closely related Middle East respiratory syndrome coronavirus (MERS-CoV) showed lack of immune response and no viral RNA detected in respiratory secretions.[16] However, one must keep in mind that SARS-CoV-2 has continued to evolve and adapt, meaning that, it is possible that more contemporary human-adapted variants will show greater potential to replicate in equids.

Molecular detection of SARS-CoV-2 in nasal secretions and/or feces of healthy horses and horses with acute onset of fever and respiratory signs has remained unsuccessful.[17,18] Even horses with close contact to SARS-CoV-2-infected keepers, track workers and riders have no to little evidence of spillover infection.[18,19] Although molecular detection of SARS-CoV-2 in respiratory secretions is limited to a short shedding period, especially in silent shedders, serology is more sensitive at capturing past-exposure. A recent serologic survey from China did not find antibodies specific to SARS-CoV-2 from healthy horses.[20] This was in sharp contrast to a study evaluating silent transmission of SARS-CoV-2 between racetrack workers with asymptomatic COVID-19 and racing thoroughbred horses.[18] This study detected specific antibodies to SARS-CoV-2 in 35/587 (5.9%) racing horses. Current CDC guidelines recommend that owners with SARS-CoV-2 avoid any close contact with their animals, including equids. A recent study documented seroconversion in one of 2 horses with direct contact to an individual (horse owner) with clinical COVID-19.[19] None of the 2 horses had detectable SARS-CoV-2 in nasal secretions, blood, and feces.

Although horses are apparently susceptible to SARS-CoV-2 and are likely to become infected through spillover from COVID-19 individuals, horses are unlikely to contribute to the spread of SARS-CoV-2. However, it is important to continue to monitor possible human-to-horse transmission, especially with the emergence of highly transmissible SARS-CoV-2 variants,[21] and to recommend that COVID-19 individuals avoid close contact with companion animals (dogs, cats, ferrets, horses).

EQUINE CORONAVIRUS
Cause

Coronaviruses are single-stranded, positive-sense, nonsegmented, enveloped RNA viruses responsible for organ-specific syndromes in a variety of mammalian and avian species.[22] The family *Coronaviridae* is subdivided in 2 subfamilies, *Torovirinae* and *Coronavirinae*, with the latter subfamily containing 4 genera defined by serologic cross-reactivity and genetic differences: *Alphacoronavirus*, *Betacoronavirus*, *Deltacoronavirus*, and *Gammacoronavirus*.[23] The *Betacoronavirus* genera is further divided into 5 subgenera (*Sarbecovirus*, *Embecovirus*, *Merbecovirus*, *Nobecovirus*, and *Hibecovirus*).[24] Equine coronavirus (ECoV) belongs to the *Embecovirus* subgenera and is phylogenetically related to bovine coronavirus (BCoV), human OC43 and HKU1 coronaviruses, canine respiratory coronavirus, mouse hepatitis virus and sialodacryoadenitis virus coronavirus OC43, and porcine hemagglutinating encephalomyelitis virus.

Table 1
Studies documenting the susceptibility of equids to severe acute respiratory syndrome coronavirus-2

Study Type	Equid (Number)	Outcome	References
Experimental infection	Horse (1)	No molecular detection of SARS-CoV-2 in nasal secretions and feces and no virus isolation from respiratory tissues	Bosco-Lauth et al,[15] 2021
Direct contact to breeders/keepers with COVID-19	Horse (34)	No detection of SARS-CoV-2 in respiratory secretions and/or feces	Cerino et al,[17] 2021
Horses with acute onset of fever and respiratory signs	Horse (667)	No detection of SARS-CoV-2 in nasal secretions	Lawton et al,[18] 2022
Serology healthy horses from China	Horse (18)	No specific antibodies against SARS-CoV-2 detected	Deng et al,[20] 2020
Serology racing horses in contact with COVID-19 track workers	Horse (587)	Antibodies against SARS-CoV-2 detected in 35/587 horses (5.9%)	Lawton et al,[18] 2022
Healthy horses in contact with COVID-19 horse owner	Horse (2)	No detection of SARS-CoV-2 in nasal secretions, blood and feces, 1 horse seroconverted against SARS-CoV-2	Pusterla et al,[19] 2022

SARS-CoV-2 belongs to the *Sarbecovirus* subgenera, whereas MERS-CoV belongs to the *Merbecovirus* subgenera.[24]

Partial and complete genome sequences from a small number of ECoV isolates from Japan, the United States, and Europe has shown high level of sequence homology ranging between 97.2% and 99.6%.[25–31] One recent report identified a novel ECoV variant from the small intestinal samples collected from 2 donkey foals with diarrhea.[32] Bioinformatic analyses showed that the novel ECoV variant shared the highest sequence identity of 97.05% with the first identified ECoV strain—NC99.[25,32] The genetic database will likely expand in the next few years as more isolates are been sequenced. This information is important in order to understand the virus at the molecular level, determine possible virulence factors, and help develop future diagnostic and preventive tools.

Epidemiology

Unfortunately, little is known about the epidemiology of ECoV, as most studies have focused on individual outbreak reports. Until the early 2010s, ECoV was considered one of many enteric pathogens associated with foal diarrhea. ECoV was first recognized as an enteric pathogen of adult horses by Oue and collaborators.[26] Since then, ECoV has been recognized as an emerging virus from adult horses with fever and enteric signs in Japan, the United States, and Europe.[26–31,33–37] ECoV has also been reported in healthy adult horses from the United States, Saudi Arabia, and Oman.[38,39]

Available demographic information has been retrieved from diagnostic laboratories showing that the overall number of ECoV positive fecal samples by quantitative PCR (qPCR) has gradually increased since the introduction of the testing in 2012 (Real-time PCR Research and Diagnostics Core Facility, University of California, Davis, USA). The increasing frequency of qPCR-positive feces likely relates to greater awareness and testing availability. It is interesting to notice that submissions from ECoV qPCR-positive cases originate from all the lower 48 states of the United States. There is also an apparent seasonality to ECoV qPCR-positive cases with a higher detection rate during the colder months of the year (**Fig. 1**),[27,40] which is similar to the seasonal disease pattern seen with the closely related BCoV.[41]

Outbreaks and individual cases of ECoV in adult horses have predominantly been reported in racing, pleasure, and show horses, and less frequently in breeding stocks. Although age-susceptibility has been recognized for many animal and human corona-viruses, one hypothesis for the apparent low frequency of clinical ECoV cases in breeding equids is that ECoV is more likely to circulate between susceptible young and adult equids at breeding farms, leading to continuous silent exposure and protection against clinical disease. However, observational exceptions are always present with biological processes and ECoV is no exception. There is one case report on an ECoV outbreak at a large American miniature horse-breeding farm with 17% of breeding animals showing clinical disease.[36]

Prevalence factors associated with seropositivity to ECoV have been studied on 5247 healthy adult horses originating from 18 states in the United States (**Table 2**).[42] A total of 504/5247 horses (9.6%) was tested seropositive to ECoV using an S1-based enzyme-linked immunosorbent assay (ELISA). Geographic origin (Midwestern regions), breed (draft breed), and use (ranch/farm use, breeding use) displayed the highest odds ratio of seroprevalence. Although breed predisposition to ECoV infection has not been determined, it is interesting to note that the initial and subsequent outbreaks from Japan all occurred in racing draft horses.[26,28] Another study evaluated the risk of exposure to ECoV in 333 apparently healthy horses from 29 farms throughout Israel using an S1-based ELISA (see **Table 2**).[43] A total of 41

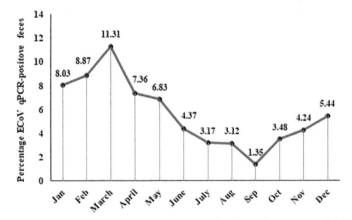

Fig. 1. Monthly distribution of ECoV qPCR-positive fecal samples among all fecal samples submitted to a private diagnostic laboratory in the United States. The data encompasses the time frame from January 2012 to May 2022.

Table 2
Seroprevalence and risk factors for equine coronavirus documented in populations of healthy adult horses in the United States and Israel

Population	Seroprevalence	Country	Risk Factors	References
Healthy horses (n = 5247)	9.6%	United States	Midwestern regions ($P = .008$) Draft horse breed ($P = .003$) Ranch/farm use ($P = .034$) Breeding use ($P = .016$)	Kooijman et al,[42] 2017
Healthy horses (n = 333)	12.3%	Israel	Northern regions ($P < .001$)	Schvartz et al,[43] 2021

out of 333 horses (12.3%) were seropositive. The ECoV seropositive horses originated from 17/29 farms (58.6%), and the seroprevalence per farm ranged from 0% to 37.5%. The only factor found to be significantly associated with ECoV exposure in the multivariable model was the geographic area, with a higher seroprevalence in horses residing in central Israel than in horses from the north or south. Longitudinal epidemiologic studies are greatly needed in order to better understand and define risk factors associated with ECoV infection in adult equids.

Clinical Disease

In field outbreaks, the morbidity rates for ECoV infections in adult horses have been reported to range from 10% to 83%.[26–28,31,32] Fatalities are rare but have been associated with disruption of the gastrointestinal mucosal barrier leading to septicemia, endotoxemia, and hyperammonemia-associated encephalopathy.[33,44]

The predominant clinical signs associated with ECoV in adult horses are nonspecific and include anorexia, lethargy, and fever ($\geq 38.6°C$; **Fig. 2, Table 3**).[26–28,31,33,34,36,37,40,45,46] Although ECoV is an enteric virus, changes in fecal character (diarrhea to soft formed feces) and/or colic are not consistently observed, findings that often challenge equine practitioners into including ECoV as a differential diagnosis. Horses with ECoV infection can sometimes develop acute neurologic signs consistent with encephalopathy and are characterized by severe lethargy, head pressing, ataxia, proprioceptive deficits, recumbency, nystagmus, and seizures.[27,33] It is speculated that the acute encephalopathic signs are caused by hyperammonemia, secondary to disruption of the gastrointestinal barrier.[44]

One must keep in mind that most ECoV infections presenting to equine veterinarians may be mild and often self-limiting, requiring minimal to no medical care. However, horses with marked to severe systemic signs are often referred to equine veterinary hospitals and the severity of clinical disease may easily mimic other gastrointestinal diseases. In a retrospective case series of 33 adult horses testing qPCR-positive for ECoV in feces, the presenting complaints were fever (83%), anorexia (47%), and colic (43%).[40] When the hospitalized horses with qPCR-positive ECoV feces were compared with a cohort of horses with fever and/or loose manure that tested qPCR-negative for ECoV infection, presenting complaints were similar.[40] Twenty-seven ECoV qPCR-positive horses were hospitalized for a median of 5 days with 26/27 (96%) surviving to discharge.[40] Another study compared clinical features of ECoV infection with enteric salmonellosis and found that the clinical signs of fever and colic were similar between the 2 groups.[45] Out of 8 horses classified as ECoV-

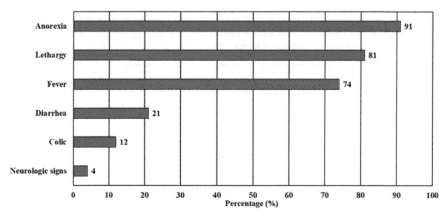

Fig. 2. Compilation of clinical signs observed from 101 adult horses with clinical ECoV infection (Pusterla, personal communication). Fever was defined as a rectal temperature ≥38.6°C. Neurologic signs were consistent with encephalopathy and included aimless wandering, circling, head pressing, recumbence, and seizure.

positive, all survived; however, 1 horse developed clinical signs consistent with laminitis.[45] Although most clinical ECoV infections are associated with outbreaks, some present as individual cases. A recent retrospective case series, including 5 horses with ECoV infection that were not associated with an outbreak, reported that anorexia and fever were observed in all horses and that 4 of 5 horses had moderate-to-severe diarrhea.[46] Patients were hospitalized for a median of 5 days and all survived to discharge. Collectively, the various case series using hospitalized horses have shown that clinical signs were not specific for ECoV and often similar to other enteric infectious diseases. However, the outcome of ECoV is favorable with the majority of the hospitalized horses surviving to discharge.

Experimental studies have shown that young and adult horses can successfully become infected with ECoV through the feco-oral route.[47–49] Because of the difficulty of growing ECoV in vitro, all experimental challenges used feces from naturally infected animals. Collectively, these studies have shown that most infected horses develop mild and self-limiting clinical signs consistent with anorexia, fever, and changes in fecal character (**Table 4**). Blood tests showed leukopenia and/or lymphopenia in approximately 50% of the infected horses, which is consistent with hematological changes observed in naturally occurring cases of ECoV infection. ECoV was detected in the feces of all experimentally infected horse via qPCR, and nasal secretions and whole blood tested occasionally qPCR-positive for ECoV. While a qPCR-positive blood sample is consistent with viremia, it could not be determined if qPCR-positive nasal secretions were due to nasal replication and shedding of the virus, from environmental contamination from the feces, or from both sources. Although experimental infections with ECoV have only been attempted in a small number of horses, it seems that clinical disease, although mild, can be consistently reproduced, making the model suitable to study the pathogenesis and the immunity of ECoV.

Diagnosis

Diagnosing ECoV infection can be challenging, especially in horses lacking specific enteric signs. The diagnosis can be supported by the presence of neutropenia and/or lymphopenia and the detection of ECoV in feces.

Table 3
Studies documenting clinical signs associated with natural equine coronavirus infection in adult horses

Population (Morbidity)	Age in Years (Median)	Country	Clinical Signs (Percentage of Reported Signs)	References
Race horses (132/600 diseased horses)	2–4	Japan	Fever, diarrhea	Oue et al,[26] 2011
Riding horses (59/165 diseased horses)	1–29 (15)	United States	Anorexia (88.1%), lethargy (77.9%), fever (72.8%), diarrhea (20.3%), colic (6.8%), neurologic signs (3.4%)	Pusterlaet al,[27] 2013
Race horses (204/650 diseased horses)	2–11 (3)	Japan	Fever (96.1%), anorexia, diarrhea (10.8%), colic (3.9%)	Oue et al,[28] 2013
Pleasure horses (7/26 diseased horses)	8–25 (18)	Switzerland	Fever (85.7%), anorexia (85.7%), cecal impaction (14.3%), diarrhea (14.3%)	Hierweger et al,[31] 2022
Miniature horses and donkey (15/27 diseased equids)	0.5–19 (6)	United States	Fever, lethargy, anorexia, colic, neurologic signs	Fielding et al,[33] 2015
Adult thoroughbred (1 diseased horse) Thoroughbred (3 diseased horses)	19 Yearling	United Kingdom	Fever, lethargy, anorexia, colic Lethargy, weight loss (concurrent larval cyathostomiasis)	Bryan et al,[34] 2019
American miniature horses (5/30 diseased horses)	0.5–12 (5)	United States	Anorexia (100%), fever (100%), lethargy, colic (40%), diarrhea (20%)	Goodrich et al,[36] 2020
Adult riding horses (15/41 diseased horses)	1–19 (10.8)	Japan	Anorexia (27%), fever (73%), lethargy (40%), diarrhea (20%)	Kambayashi et al,[37] 2021
Hospitalized adult horses (33 diseased horses)	2–37 (11)	United States	Fever (83%), anorexia (47%), colic (43%), lethargy (27%), diarrhea (3%), foot soreness (3)	Berryhill et al,[40] 2019
Hospitalized adult horses (8 diseased horses)	3–16 (6.5)	United States	Fever (50%), lethargy (25%), anorexia (12.5%), colic (12.5%), diarrhea (25%)	Manship et al,[45] 2019
Hospitalized adult horses (5 diseased horses)	8–13 (9)	United States	Fever (100%), anorexia (100%), lethargy (60%), colic (40%), diarrhea (20%)	Mattei et al,[46] 2020

Table 4
Studies documenting clinical, hematological and laboratory findings associated with experimental equine coronavirus infection in young and adult horses

Population (Number of Horses)	Clinical Signs	Blood Work	Molecular Testing	Serology	References
9–10-month-old draft horses (3)	Fever (2), anorexia (2), pasty feces (2)	Leukopenia/lymphopenia (1), elevated SAA (2)	ECoV RNA in feces (3), nasal secretions (3), and blood (2)	Seroconversion (3)	Nemoto et al,[47] 2014
Adult horses (8)	Gastrointestinal hypermotility (7), loose manure (7), fever (1)	Lymphopenia (4)	ECoV RNA in feces (8), nasal secretions (4), and blood (1)	Seroconversion (4)	Schaefer et al,[48] 2018
Yearling Thoroughbred horses (4)	Fever (2)	Not applicable	ECoV RNA in feces (4), nasal secretions (3), and blood (2)	Not applicable	Kambayashi et al,[49] 2022

The number of horses for each of the parameters is listed in parenthesis.

Hematological findings of ECoV infections are generally consistent with a viral hemogram characterized by leukopenia due to neutropenia and/or lymphopenia. In a review of 35 cell blood counts from horses with natural ECoV infection supported through qPCR detection of coronavirus in feces, 74% of diseased horsed showed leukopenia, 66% neutrophilia, and 72% lymphopenia (**Fig. 3**). It is, however, important to keep in mind that approximately 10% of horses with ECoV infection display an unremarkable hemogram. Hematological abnormalities are expected to resolve within 5 to 7 days as long as no complications associated with the disruption of the gastrointestinal barrier occur. Less consistent hematological abnormalities can include the presence of band neutrophils, monocytosis and leukocytosis due to neutrophilia and monocytosis during the recovery period. When 8 clinical cases of ECoV infection were compared with 12 horses with enteric salmonellosis, neutrophil count was decreased in both groups but was not significantly different.[45] Further, in a case series of 33 horses with ECoV infection seen at a veterinary hospital, ECoV qPCR-positive horses had lower white blood cells (range 680–16,200/μL, median 3000/μL), neutrophil counts (150–14,400/μL, median 1250/μL), and lymphocyte counts (420–3470/μL, median 860/μL) when compared with ECoV qPCR-negative horses.[40]

Serum biochemistry profiles may be unremarkable; however, abnormalities in ECoV-infected horses have been reported and include electrolyte derangements, hyperbilirubinemia, hyperglycemia, hyperlipidemia, hypoproteinemia, increased muscle enzymes, and azotemia.[40] ECoV infection with concurrent signs of encephalopathy has been linked to hyperammonemia. A recent ECoV case series reported on 1 horse with severe hyperammonemia (677 μmol/L; reference interval ≤60 μmol/L) with encephalopathic signs that subsequently died.[33] Hyperammonemia associated with ECoV infection is likely due to increased ammonia production within or absorption from the gastrointestinal tract due to gastrointestinal barrier breakdown. An increase in enteric ammonia production could also be the result of bacterial microbiome changes associated with ECoV infection.

It is only in recent years that the diagnostics for ECoV have markedly improved with the use of qPCR. The limitation of historic detection modalities, such as negative stain electron microscopy (EM) or antigen-capture ELISA, is that they are not sensitive enough when viral particles are not present in sufficient numbers. The biological sample of choice to support an ECoV diagnosis is feces or rectal swabs. Previous work has shown that molecular assays are rapid, cost-effective, sensitive, and specific for ECoV.[27,36,50] Unfortunately, no study has compared the various molecular techniques (qPCR vs RT loop-mediated isothermal amplification) and their superior sensitivity to negative stain EM or antigen-capture ELISA. Although the detection of ECoV in the feces of diseased horses is highly suggestive of infection, one must keep in mind that 4% to 83% of horses can remain subclinically infected during an ECoV outbreak.[27,33,36,37] Viral kinetics of ECoV in feces from experimentally infected horses have shown that horses begin to shed detectable ECoV RNA in their feces at 3 or 4 days postinfection and continue shedding virus until 12 or 14 days postinfection.[47–49] Peak ECoV shedding is consistently seen on day 3 to 4 following the development of clinical disease (**Fig. 4**). Average length of ECoV RNA detection following onset of natural infection ranges from 3 to 9 days, however, naturally infected horses have been shown to sporadically shed ECoV RNA in feces up to 98 days.[27,33,36,37] Although additional biological samples such as whole blood (viremia) and nasal secretions (shedding) have tested qPCR-positive for ECoV in experimentally[47–49] and naturally[29,51,52] occurring infections, these sample types do not consistently test positive and should not be used to support a diagnosis of ECoV infection. The molecular detection of ECoV can be challenging, especially during peracute disease when

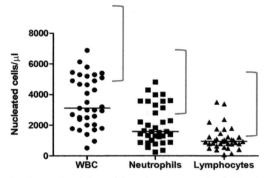

Fig. 3. White blood cell, neutrophil, and lymphocyte count of 35 adult horses with suspected ECoV infection. The results are expressed as individual values. Median values are represented by horizontal bars. Red brackets represent normal reference ranges for each cellular fraction displayed (WBC 5000–11,600/μL; neutrophil count 2600–6800/μL; lymphocyte count 1600–5800 μL).

diseased horses experience gastrointestinal stasis due to colic and/or there are not enough viral particles in the feces to be detected. Recommendations are to repeat testing of fecal matter in a suspected index case at a later time point or collect multiple samples for pooled testing. Further, it has been the author's experience that ECoV-infected horses presenting with systemic clinical signs such as fever, lethargy, and anorexia are more likely to be tested for respiratory pathogens through respiratory secretions than enteric pathogens through feces. In order to speed up diagnostic turn-around-time, one should consider submitting both, nasal secretions and feces, in adult horses with acute onset of systemic signs in order to test for selected respiratory and enteric pathogens or stage the testing to the more likely cause. This process will speed up the analysis because additional samples (ie, feces) have already been shipped to the laboratory and are available for ECoV testing.

Serology has been established and validated for ECoV and is available in research laboratories mostly to document seroconversion in experimentally infected horses or study the epidemiology of ECoV in various horse populations.[26,28,42,43,47,48,53,54] Serology can be used to retrospectively establish recent infection using acute and convalescent serum samples and documenting either seroconversion or increase in serum titers.

Necropsy cases of suspected enteritis should have feces or gastrointestinal content tested by qPCR for ECoV and other gastrointestinal infectious agents. Further, formalin-fixed intestinal tissue samples can also be tested by immunochemistry and direct fluorescent antibody testing using BCoV reagents.[44]

Pathogenesis

Following an incubation period of 48 to 72 hours, most horses infected with ECoV develop a self-limiting enteritis, which generally resolves with minimal supportive care. In most clinical adult horses, ECoV is the only pathogen detected in the feces of affected horses, suggesting a unique pathogenicity.[27,28,40] However, little is known about the pathogenesis of ECoV, other than its tropism to enterocytes.[55,56] A recent case series reported on the pathologic condition of ECoV infection in 3 naturally infected equids with sudden death.[44] Gross and histologic findings were consistent with severe diffuse necrotizing enteritis, characterized by marked villus attenuation,

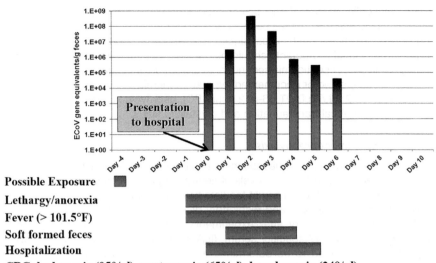

Possible Exposure

Lethargy/anorexia

Fever (> 101.5°F)

Soft formed feces

Hospitalization

CBC: leukopenia (950/µl), neutropenia (650/µl), lymphopenia (240/µl)

Fig. 4. Diagram showing temporal clinical signs and fecal shedding of ECoV in an adult horse presented to a referring hospital because of anorexia, lethargy, and fever.

epithelial cell necrosis in the tips of the villi, neutrophilic and fibrin extravasation into the small intestinal lumen, as well as crypt necrosis, microthrombosis, and hemorrhage. In these 3 necropsied cases, ECoV was detected by qPCR in intestinal tissue, gastrointestinal content, and/or feces. Further, coronavirus antigen was detected by immunohistochemistry and/or direct fluorescent antibody testing in the small intestine of all cases. In comparison to BCoV, there is no evidence that ECoV has respiratory tropism based on the lack of respiratory signs in affected equids and histologic changes in horses undergoing necropsy.[57] The lack of respiratory tropism is supported by a recent experimental study, which showed that in only 1 out of 4 horses, ECoV was detected in the lungs by qPCR but not by in situ hybridization.[49] Apparently, lung cells themselves were not susceptible to ECoV and qPCR-positive lung tissue was caused by viremia.[49]

One rare complication of clinical ECoV has been the development of often-fatal encephalopathy, suspected to occur secondary to hyperammonemia.[33] In the case series reporting on the pathologic condition of ECoV infection in 3 naturally infected equids, one of them displayed hyperammonemic encephalopathy with Alzheimer type II astrocytosis throughout the cerebral cortex, suggesting a strong association between ECoV necrotizing enteritis, hyperammonemia and the development of encephalopathy.[44]

Therapeutic Strategies

Most horses with clinical ECoV infection recover in a few days with little supportive to no treatment at all. Horses showing persistent elevated rectal temperature affecting their appetite and attitude have been treated with antipyretic (dipyrone at 30 mg/kg body weight [BWT] q12–24 hours intravenous [IV]) or anti-inflammatory drugs (flunixin meglumine [0.5–1.1 mg/kg BWT q12–24 hours IV or per os [PO]; phenylbutazone [2–4 mg/kg BWT q12–24 hours IV or PO]; firocoxib [0.1 mg/kg BWT q24 hours PO or 0.09 mg/kg BWT q24 hours IV]) for 24 to 48 hours, as long as they stay hydrated.

Horses with colic, persistent anorexia, and/or diarrhea have been treated more intensively with fluid and electrolytes per nasogastric intubation or intravenous administration of polyionic fluids until clinical signs have resolved. Additionally, antimicrobials and gastrointestinal protectants should be considered in horses developing signs of endotoxemia and/or septicemia secondary to disruption of the gastrointestinal barrier. Horses with suspected or documented hyperammonemia should be treated with oral lactulose (0.1–0.2 mL/kg BWT q6-q12 hours PO), neomycin sulfate (4–8 mg/kg BWT q8 hours PO), or fecal transfaunation and crystalloid fluids.

Immunity and Immunoprophylaxis

Less is known about the immune responses and immune protection against ECoV. For the closely-related BCoV, serum levels of neutralizing and HI antibody from naturally infected calves and cattle arriving at feedlots have been shown to correlate with protection against both, enteric and respiratory disease.[58-61] Further, cattle that recovered from winter dysentery after experimental infection with BCoV maintained a very long-lasting BCoV-specific serum (IgA and IgG) and local (IgA) antibody response.[62] It will need to be determined if certain levels of antibodies and what type of specific immune response correlates with protection against ECoV.

Immunization strategies have been best described in cattle for the prevention of winter dysentery infection using commercially available BCoV vaccines. Due to the close genetic homology of ECoV with BCoV, serologic responses to BCoV vaccines have recently been investigated in horses. One study used a killed-adjuvanted BCoV vaccine in 6 healthy yearling horses and reported a measurable serologic response in all horses following the administration of 2 vaccines given 28 days apart.[63] A second study investigated the safety, humoral response, and viral shedding in horses inoculated either orally, intranasally, or intrarectally with a commercially available modified-live BCoV vaccine.[64] The results of that study showed that the modified-live BCoV was safe to administer to horses through various routes, caused minimal virus shedding and resulted in detectable antibodies to BCoV in 27% of the vaccinates. Collectively, these 2 BCoV vaccines, while showing measurable antibody responses to BCoV, cannot be recommended at the present time due to the lack of efficacy data.

Control Strategies

The cornerstone of ECoV prevention resides in strict biosecurity measures aimed at reducing the risk of introducing and disseminating ECoV on equine premises. It is important to be vigilant when working-up horses presenting with fever, anorexia, and lethargy, with or without concurrent enteric signs. Such horses should be isolated until ECoV, as well as other potential infectious pathogens, have been ruled in or out. ECoV qPCR-positive horses should be isolated and stable-mates or herd-mates closely monitored until the outcome of past-exposure has been determined. Outbreaks of ECoV are generally short lasting, especially when strict biosecurity measures have been followed, and quarantine can routinely be lifted 2 to 3 weeks following the resolution of clinical signs in the last affected horse.

Coronaviruses are susceptible to heat, detergents, and disinfectants such as sodium hypochlorite, povidone iodine, 70% ethanol, glutaraldehyde, quaternary ammonium compounds, phenolic compounds, formaldehyde, peroxymonosulfate, and accelerated hydrogen peroxide.[65-68] Moreover, coronaviruses have been reported to survive well at low temperatures and high relative humidity. Their survival on surfaces is also long, up to 120 hours and even longer in organic medium such as feces, urine, and wastewater.[69-72]

SUMMARY

As incidental hosts, horses are unlikely to contribute to the spread of SARS-CoV-2. Rare infections of SARS-CoV-2 have been reported in equids, thought to occur secondary to the spillover of SARS-CoV-2 from symptomatic or asymptomatic COVID-19 individuals. ECoV has emerged as an enteric pathogen of adult horses in recent years and has been reported in Japan, Europe, and the United States. There are increasing reports of the disease, arising from increased awareness in the field and the availability of diagnostic tests for detecting ECoV in feces of affected horses. Clinical presentation of ECoV infection is often limited to systemic signs such as fever, lethargy, and anorexia, although enteric signs are present in less than 20% of infected cases. Although blood tests may suggest a viral infection (lymphopenia and neutropenia), laboratory diagnosis is supported by the detection of ECoV in feces using qPCR. ECoV infection is often self-limiting, requiring little to no supportive treatment. Although no vaccine is available now, prevention of ECoV infection is best achieved through routine management practices aimed at reducing the likelihood of introducing and disseminating ECoV at any horse-based premise as well as the timely isolation of horses with suspected clinical ECoV infection.

CLINICS CARE POINTS

- Equids are deadend hosts to SARS-CoV-2 and do not contribute to the COVID-19 pandemic.
- ECoV often causes only systemic clincial signs in adult horses.
- ECoV is diagnosed via the molecular detection of ECoV in feces.
- ECoV is often a self-limiting disease requiring little to no medical treatment.

DISCLOSURE

The author has nothing to disclose.

REFERENCES

1. Jo WK, de Oliveira-Filho EF, Rasche A, et al. Potential zoonotic sources of SARS-CoV-2 infections. Transbound Emerg Dis 2021;68:1824–34.
2. Hobbs EC, Reid TJ. Animals and SARS-CoV-2: Species susceptibility and viral transmission in experimental and natural conditions, and the potential implications for community transmission. Transbound Emerg Dis 2021;68:1850–67.
3. Murphy HL, Ly H. Understanding the prevalence of SARS-CoV-2 (COVID-19) exposure in companion, captive, wild, and farmed animals. Virulence 2021;12:2777–86.
4. do Vale B, Lopes AP, Fontes MDC, et al. Bats, pangolins, minks and other animals - villains or victims of SARS-CoV-2? Vet Res Commun 2021;45:1–19.
5. Pickering BS, Smith G, Pinette MM, et al. Susceptibility of domestic swine to experimental infection with severe acute respiratory syndrome coronavirus 2. Emerg Infect Dis 2021;27:104–12.
6. Patterson EI, Elia G, Grassi A, et al. Evidence of exposure to SARS-CoV-2 in cats and dogs from households in Italy. Nat Commun 2020;11:6231.

7. Sailleau C, Dumarest M, Vanhomwegen J, et al. First detection and genome sequencing of SARS-CoV-2 in an infected cat in France. Transbound Emerg Dis 2020;67:2324–8.

8. Barrs VR, Peiris M, Tam KWS, et al. SARS-CoV-2 in quarantined domestic cats from COVID-19 households or close contacts, Hong Kong, China. Emerg Infect Dis 2020;26:3071–4.

9. Calvet GA, Pereira SA, Ogrzewalska M, et al. Investigation of SARS-CoV-2 infection in dogs and cats of humans diagnosed with COVID-19 in Rio de Janeiro, Brazil. PLoS ONE 2021;16:e0250853.

10. Ruiz-Arrondo I, Portillo A, Palomar AM, et al. Detection of SARS-CoV-2 in pets living with COVID-19 owners diagnosed during the COVID-19 lockdown in Spain: A case of an asymptomatic cat with SARS-CoV-2 in Europe. Transbound Emerg Dis 2021;68:973–6.

11. Hamer SA, Pauvolid-Corrêa A, Zecca IB, et al. SARS-CoV-2 infections and viral isolations among serially tested cats and dogs in households with infected owners in Texas, USA. Viruses 2021;13:938.

12. Hossain MG, Javed A, Akter S, et al. SARS-CoV-2 host diversity: An update of natural infections and experimental evidence. J Microbiol Immunol Infect 2021; 54:175–81.

13. Damas J, Hughes GM, Keough KC, et al. Broad host range of SARS-CoV-2 predicted by comparative and structural analysis of ACE2 in vertebrates. Proc Natl Acad Sci U S A 2020;117:22311–22.

14. Liu Y, Hu G, Wang Y, et al. Functional and genetic analysis of viral receptor ACE2 orthologs reveals a broad potential host range of SARS-CoV-2. Proc Natl Acad Sci U S A 2021;118. e2025373118.

15. Bosco-Lauth AM, Walker A, Guilbert L, et al. Susceptibility of livestock to SARS-CoV-2 infection. Emerg Microbes Infect 2021;10:2199–201.

16. Vergara-Alert J, van den Brand JM, Widagdo W, et al. Livestock susceptibility to infection with Middle East respiratory syndrome coronavirus. Emerg Infect Dis 2017;23:232–40.

17. Cerino P, Buonerba C, Brambilla G, et al. No detection of SARS-CoV-2 in animals exposed to infected keepers: results of a COVID-19 surveillance program. Future Sci OA 2021;7:FSO711.

18. Lawton KOY, Arthur RM, Moeller BC, et al. Investigation of the role of healthy and sick equids in the COVID-19 pandemic through serological and molecular testing. Animals 2022;12:614.

19. Pusterla N, Chaillon A, Ignacio C, et al. SARS-CoV-2 seroconversion in an adult horse with direct contact to a COVID-19 individual. Viruses 2022;14:1047.

20. Deng J, Jin Y, Liu Y, et al. Serological survey of SARS-CoV-2 for experimental, domestic, companion and wild animals excludes intermediate hosts of 35 different species of animals. Transbound Emerg Dis 2020;67:1745–9.

21. Boehm E, Kronig I, Neher RA, et al. Novel SARS-CoV-2 variants: the pandemics within the pandemic. Clin Microbiol Infect 2021;27:1109–17.

22. Wege H, Siddell S, Ter Meulen V. The biology and pathogenesis of coronaviruses. Curr Top Microbiol Immunol 1982;99:165–200.

23. Woo PC, Lau SK, Lam CS, et al. Discovery of seven novel mammalian and avian coronaviruses in the genus deltacoronavirus supports bat coronaviruses as the gene source of alphacoronavirus and betacoronavirus and avian coronaviruses as the gene source of Gammacoronavirus and Deltacoronavirus. J Virol 2012; 86:3995–4008.

24. Dhama K, Khan S, Tiwari R, et al. Coronavirus Disease 2019-COVID-19. Clin Microbiol Rev 2020;33:e00028.
25. Zhang J, Guy JS, Snijder EJ, et al. Genomic characterization of equine coronavirus. Virology 2007;369:92–104.
26. Oue Y, Ishihara R, Edamatsu H, et al. Isolation of an equine coronavirus from adult horses with pyrogenic and enteric disease and its antigenic and genomic characterization in comparison with the NC99 strain. Vet Microbiol 2011;150:41–8.
27. Pusterla N, Mapes S, Wademan C, et al. Emerging outbreaks associated with equine coronavirus in adult horses. Vet Microbiol 2013;162:228–31.
28. Oue Y, Morita Y, Kondo T, et al. Epidemic of equine coronavirus at Obihiro Racecourse, Hokkaido, Japan in 2012. Vet Med Sci 2013;75:1261–5.
29. Miszczak F, Tesson V, Kin N, et al. First detection of equine coronavirus (ECoV) in Europe. Vet Microbiol 2014;171:206–9.
30. Nemoto M, Oue Y, Murakami S, et al. Complete genome analysis of equine coronavirus isolated in Japan. Arch Virol 2015;160:2903–6.
31. Hierweger MM, Remy-Wohlfender F, Franzen J, et al. Outbreak of equine coronavirus disease in adult horses, Switzerland 2021. Transbound Emerg Dis 2022;69:1691–4.
32. Qi PF, Gao XY, Ji JK, et al. Identification of a recombinant equine coronavirus in donkey, China. Emerg Microbes Infect 2022;11:1010–3.
33. Fielding CL, Higgins JK, Higgins JC, et al. Disease associated with equine coronavirus infection and high case fatality rate. J Vet Intern Med 2015;29:307–10.
34. Bryan J, Marr CM, Mackenzie CJ, et al. Detection of equine coronavirus in horses in the United Kingdom. Vet Rec 2019;184:123.
35. Nemoto M, Schofield W, Cullinane A. The first detection of equine coronavirus in adult horses and foals in Ireland. Viruses 2019;11:946.
36. Goodrich EL, Mittel LD, Glaser A, et al. Novel findings from a beta coronavirus outbreak on an American Miniature Horse breeding farm in upstate New York. Equine Vet Educ 2020;32:150–4.
37. Kambayashi Y, Bannai H, Tsujimura K, et al. Outbreak of equine coronavirus infection among riding horses in Tokyo, Japan. Comp Immunol Microbiol Infect Dis 2021;77:101668.
38. Hemida MG, Chu DKW, Perera RAPM, et al. Coronavirus infections in horses in Saudi Arabia and Oman. Transbound Emerg Dis 2017;64:2093–103.
39. Stout AE, Hofmar-Glennon HG, André NM, et al. Infectious disease surveillance of apparently healthy horses at a multi-day show using a novel nanoscale real-time PCR panel. Vet Diagn Invest 2021;33:80–6.
40. Berryhill EH, Magdesian KG, Aleman M, et al. Clinical presentation, diagnostic findings, and outcome of adult horses with equine coronavirus infection at a veterinary teaching hospital: 33 cases (2012-2018). Vet J 2019;248:95–100.
41. Zhu Q, Li B, Sun D. Advances in bovine coronavirus epidemiology. Viruses 2022;14:1109.
42. Kooijman LJ, James K, Mapes SM, et al. Seroprevalence and risk factors for infection with equine coronavirus in healthy horses in the USA. Vet J 2017;220:91–4.
43. Schvartz G, Tirosh-Levy S, Barnum S, et al. Seroprevalence and risk factors for exposure to equine coronavirus in apparently healthy horses in Israel. Animals 2021;11:894.

44. Giannitti F, Diab S, Mete A, et al. Necrotizing enteritis and hyperammonemic encephalopathy associated with equine coronavirus infection in equids. Vet Pathol 2015;52:1148–56.
45. Manship AJ, Blikslager AT, Elfenbein JR. Disease features of equine coronavirus and enteric salmonellosis are similar in horses. J Vet Intern Med 2019;33:912–7.
46. Mattei DN, Kopper JJ, Sanz MG. Equine coronavirus-associated colitis in horses: a retrospective study. J Equine Vet Sci 2020;87:102906.
47. Nemoto M, Oue Y, Morita Y, et al. Experimental inoculation of equine coronavirus into Japanese draft horses. Arch Virol 2014;159:3329–34.
48. Schaefer E, Harms C, Viner M, et al. Investigation of an experimental infection model of equine coronavirus in adult horses. J Vet Intern Med 2018;32:2099–104.
49. Kambayashi Y, Kishi D, Ueno T, et al. Distribution of equine coronavirus RNA in the intestinal and respiratory tracts of experimentally infected horses. Arch Virol 2022;167:1611–8.
50. Nemoto M, Morita Y, Niwa H, et al. Rapid detection of equine coronavirus by reverse transcription loop-mediated isothermal amplification. J Virol Methods 2015;215-216:13–6.
51. Pusterla N, Holzenkaempfer N, Mapes S, et al. Prevalence of equine coronavirus in nasal secretions from horses with fever and upper respiratory tract infection. Vet Rec 2015;177:289.
52. Pusterla N, James K, Mapes S, et al. Frequency of molecular detection of equine coronavirus in faeces and nasal secretions in 277 horses with acute onset of fever. Vet Rec 2019;184:385.
53. Kooijman LJ, Mapes SM, Pusterla N. Development of an equine coronavirus-specific enzyme-linked immunosorbent assay to determine serologic responses in naturally infected horses. J Vet Diagn Invest 2016;28:414–8.
54. Zhao S, Smits C, Schuurman N, et al. Development and validation of a S1 protein-based ELISA for the specific detection of antibodies against equine coronavirus. Viruses 2019;11:1109.
55. Davis E, Rush BR, Cox J, et al. Neonatal enterocolitis associated with coronavirus infection in a foal: a case report. J Vet Diagn Invest 2000;12:153–6.
56. Guy JS, Breslin JJ, Breuhaus B, et al. Characterization of a coronavirus isolated from a diarrheic foal. J Clin Microbiol 2000;38:4523–6.
57. Park SJ, Kim GY, Choy HE, et al. Dual enteric and respiratory tropisms of winter dysentery bovine coronavirus in calves. Arch Virol 2007;152:1885–900.
58. Thomas CJ, Hoet AE, Sreevatsan S, et al. Transmission of bovine coronavirus and serologic responses in feedlot calves under field conditions. Am J Vet Res 2006;67:1412–20.
59. Heckert RA, Saif LJ, Myers GW, et al. Epidemiologic factors and isotype-specific antibody responses in serum and mucosal secretions of dairy calves with bovine coronavirus respiratory tract and enteric tract infections. Am J Vet Res 1991;52:845–51.
60. Lin X, O'reilly KL, Burrell ML, et al. Infectivity-neutralizing and hemagglutinin-inhibiting antibody responses to respiratory coronavirus infections of cattle in pathogenesis of shipping fever pneumonia. Clin Diagn Lab Immunol 2001;8:357–62.
61. Lin XQ, O'reilly KL, Storz J. Antibody responses of cattle with respiratory coronavirus infections during pathogenesis of shipping fever pneumonia are lower with antigens of enteric strains than with those of a respiratory strain. Clin Diagn Lab Immunol 2002;9:1010–3.

62. Tråvén M, Näslund K, Linde N, et al. Experimental reproduction of winter dysentery in lactating cows using BCV - comparison with BCV infection in milk-fed calves. Vet Microbiol 2001;81:127–51.
63. Nemoto M, Kanno T, Bannai H, et al. Antibody response to equine coronavirus in horses inoculated with a bovine coronavirus vaccine. J Vet Med Sci 2017;79:1889–91.
64. Prutton JSW, Barnum S, Pusterla N. Evaluation of safety, humoral immune response and faecal shedding in horses inoculated with a modified-live bovine coronavirus vaccine. Equine Vet Educ 2019;32:33–6.
65. Sattar SA, Springthorpe VS, Karim Y, et al. Chemical disinfection of non-porous inanimate surfaces experimentally contaminated with four human pathogenic viruses. Epidemiol Infect 1989;102:493–505.
66. Holtkamp DJ, Myers J, Thomas PR, et al. Efficacy of an accelerated hydrogen peroxide disinfectant to inactivate porcine epidemic diarrhea virus in swine feces on metal surfaces. Can J Vet Res 2017;81:100–7.
67. Huang YS, Bilyeu AN, Hsu WW, et al. Treatment with dry hydrogen peroxide accelerates the decay of severe acute syndrome coronavirus-2 on non-porous hard surfaces. Am J Infect Control 2021;49:1252–5.
68. Choi H, Chatterjee P, Lichtfouse E, et al. Classical and alternative disinfection strategies to control the COVID-19 virus in healthcare facilities: a review. Environ Chem Lett 2021;19:1945–51.
69. Duan SM, Zhao XS, Wen RF, et al. Stability of SARS coronavirus in human specimens and environment and its sensitivity to heating and UV irradiation. Biomed Environ Sci 2003;16:246–55.
70. Geller C, Varbanov M, Duval RE. Human coronaviruses: insights into environmental resistance and its influence on the development of new antiseptic strategies. Viruses 2012;4:3044–68.
71. Wang XW, Li JS, Jin M, et al. Study on the resistance of severe acute respiratory syndrome-associated coronavirus. J Virol Methods 2005;126:171–7.
72. Watanabe M, Ohnishi T, Arai S, et al. Survival of SARS-CoV-2 and bovine coronavirus on common surfaces of living environments. Sci Rep 2022;12:10624.

Infectious Causes of Equine Placentitis and Abortion

Rebecca E. Ruby, MSc, BVSc, Diplomate ACVP, ACVIM-LAIM*,
Jennifer G. Janes, DVM, PhD, Diplomate ACVP

KEYWORDS

- Equine • Abortion • Placentitis

KEY POINTS

- A variety of infectious etiologies can cause abortion in equines.
- Selection of the appropriate samples is crucial to determine a diagnosis in most cases.
- Complete histories and ancillary diagnostic testing in conjunction with the examination of the fetus and placenta will increase the likelihood of diagnosis.
- Not all equine causes of equine abortion have macroscopic lesions and so submission of histopathology and ancillary testing is recommended in all cases.
- Mares that have been aborted should be isolated from other mares until contagious causes of abortion have been ruled out.

INTRODUCTION

Infectious causes of equine abortion and placentitis include a variety of viral, bacterial, and fungal organisms. The prevalence of different diseases varies between years and regions, but in all cases, identification of a cause of abortion will help to determine the need for enhanced biosecurity, vaccination, or post-partum intervention. A complete examination of fetal membranes by experienced farm staff or veterinarians is recommended in all cases. When a compromised foal is born, or a fetus is aborted, then submission of the fetus and placenta to a diagnostic laboratory is most likely to yield a diagnosis. Many causes of equine abortion are considered idiopathic or due to structural abnormalities and will not be discussed here. In all cases, if sufficient tissues are submitted, infectious causes of abortion can be ruled in or out.

DISCUSSION
Placental Anatomy Overview

Horses have a diffuse, endotheliochorial placentation that attaches throughout the uterus except for the cervical star. Two structures, the chorioallantois, and allantoamnion make up the placenta. The chorionic surface is composed of microcotyledons that

Department of Veterinary Science, University of Kentucky, Veterinary Diagnostic Laboratory, 1490 Bull Lea Road, Lexington, KY 40511, USA
* Corresponding author.
E-mail address: rebecca.ruby@uky.edu

Vet Clin Equine 39 (2023) 73–88
https://doi.org/10.1016/j.cveq.2022.11.001
0749-0739/23/© 2022 Elsevier Inc. All rights reserved.
vetequine.theclinics.com

allow close apposition of blood vessels for oxygen exchange between the fetus and dam. Following 150 days of gestation, the placenta will have recognizable anatomy including the gravid, non-gravid horn, body, and cervical star. The umbilical cord should attach to the base of either uterine horn. The cervical star is an avillous region of chorioallantois that opposes the cervix. Recognition of the normal anatomy and appearance of the placenta will assist in the diagnosis of placentitis, appropriate sample selection, and early recognition of potentially infectious agents. The chorionic surface should predominantly be red and velvety due to the presence of microcotyledons (**Fig. 1**). Avillous areas may occur at the cervical star, endometrial cups, areas of endometrial cysts or places where placental folds occurred. Typically, these occupy only a small portion of the placental surface. A multitude of normal variations may occur, but when presented with an abortion or suspected placental abnormality, the authors recommend collecting all potential areas of concern for histopathologic evaluation. A list of recommended fetal tissues is provided (**Table 1**).

Viral Diseases

Equine herpesvirus

Equine herpesvirus (EHV) causes infections in horses worldwide. Subtypes 1 to 5 infect domestic horses leading to a variety of clinical presentations. The alphaherpesviruses, EHV-1 and to a lesser extent EHV-4, cause equine abortion. Abortions can be sporadic in nature or abortion storms can occur.[1] The most common route of infection is inhalation of viral particles, although direct contact with infected aborted fetuses and fetal membranes or contaminated fomites can also serve as a source.[2] Mares are the primary source of infection to young foals, thereby creating a landscape of widespread infection in young stock. Once a horse is infected, virus targets respiratory epithelium, lymphoid tissue, and circulating CD 4 and CD 8 T lymphocytes and monocytes in the bloodstream (cell-associated viremia). Virus can then be transported throughout the body. Critical to EHV pathogenesis and maintenance in the equine

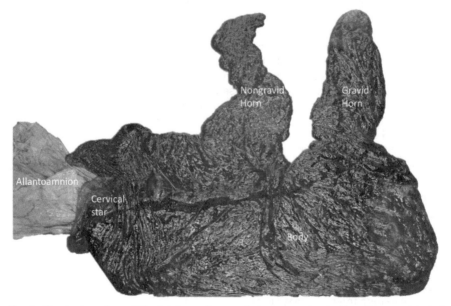

Fig. 1. Chorionic surface of the fetal membranes. Relevant anatomical locations are labeled.

Table 1
Routine tissue collection for diagnostic testing of cases of equine abortion or placentitis

Tissue of Interest	Sample Type	Test Offering[a]
• Liver, lung, spleen, adrenal gland, kidney, placenta[b]	• Fresh tissue- individually bagged, labeled and chilled	• Bacterial culture • Fungal culture • Fluorescent antibody testing • Virus isolation • PCR
• Visceral: Liver, lung, spleen, kidney, adrenal gland, heart, gastrointestinal tract (stomach, small and large intestine) and skeletal muscle • Placenta: middle of each horn, body, cervical star, amnion and umbilical cord, as well as any sites which appear abnormal	• Formalin Fixed Tissue (tissue combined in sealed contained with 10% neutral buffered formalin)	• Routine Histology • Immunohistochemistry
• Fetal heart blood • Maternal peripheral blood	• Red top (fetus and mare) • EDTA (mare)	• Serology • PCR

Note: A combination of tissues and placenta may be submitted for testing for EHV-1, leptospirosis, Equine Arteritis virus and bacterial or fungal culture. In some cases, such as an EHV-1 abortion, a respiratory swab, and EDTA blood and serum from the mare may be included.
   [a] Available testing may vary based on laboratory test offerings.
   [b] Multiple pieces of fresh and formalin fixed tissue, typically 2-3 of each, will help expedite laboratory processing.

population is the cycle of latency and reactivation after infection. Viral latency occurs within T lymphocytes and the trigeminal ganglia.[3] When reactivation occurs, whether it is due to stress, transport, corticosteroid administration or some other variable, replication of virus in the respiratory epithelium can produce a viremia leading to uterine endothelial cell infection that can result in vasculitis and transplacental spread leading to abortion.[1,4–7] Uterine endothelial cells appear to be less susceptible to viral infection early in gestation as compared with later which fits with the timing of mid-to late-term abortions or perinatal death.[7] Different strains have been found to have variable abortigenic potential.[8–11] In addition, both non-neuropathic and neuropathic strains have been found to cause abortion.[12,13]

Abortion can occur without premonitory signs and most commonly occurs as a result of EHV-1. EHV-4 causing abortion is sporadic and less common.[14] Gross lesions in aborted fetuses include subcutaneous edema, amber fluid in the thoracic and/or abdominal cavity, heavy edematous lungs that may have rib impressions and scattered 1 to 4 mm tan to gray foci on the parenchyma. Tracheal fibrin casts, few to numerous pinpoint white to gray foci scattered on the capsular surface of the liver, and petechial to ecchymotic hemorrhages can be distributed across multiple organs (**Fig. 2**). Microscopically, fetal lung lesions are composed of necrosis of bronchiolar and alveolar epithelial cells that contain acidophilic intranuclear viral inclusion bodies, mononuclear inflammation, and interlobular edema. Hepatic lesions of aborted fetuses are composed of randomly distributed lytic necrosis with viral intranuclear inclusion bodies occasionally observed in peripheral intact hepatocytes. Similar foci of necrosis are observed in the thymus, spleen, lymph nodes, adrenal gland.[15]

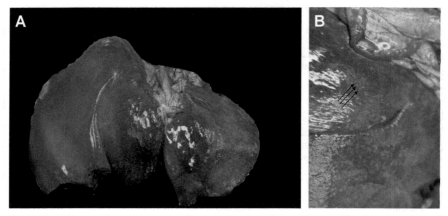

Fig. 2. Liver from a fetus with a confirmed abortion due to EHV-1. The liver is enlarged. Numerous pinpoint grey foci are scattered across all liver lobes. Figure B is higher magnification of A with several necrotic foci indicated with black arrows.

Grossly and microscopically the placenta is normal. Meconium staining of the fetal membranes, eponychium, and aspiration are compatible with fetal stress. It should be noted there is variation in which organs may be affected in aborted fetuses; therefore, complete postmortem examination or a field necropsy collecting all potentially affected tissues maximizes diagnostic value. Confirmatory testing for abortion due to EHV includes immunohistochemistry (IHC), virus isolation (VI) or polymerase chain reaction (PCR) of fetal tissues.[16,17] Optimal fetal tissues for testing include spleen, lung, thymus, and liver.

Given improved management and control measures (ie, segregation of pregnant mares from other horses, subgrouping of smaller numbers of mares, reducing stress, proper vaccination, etc.) for EHV-1 over time, "abortion storms" are not as common but can occur in the absence of these protocols.[2,17,18] Regarding vaccination, the modified live vaccine has been found to be safe to administer to pregnant mares; however, there is no label claim against abortion to EHV-1. The killed vaccines show variable data as to whether they confer protection against abortion.[19–21]

Equine viral arteritis

Equine viral arteritis (EVA) is a worldwide disease caused by the single-stranded, positive sense, RNA equine arteritis virus (EAV) within the *Arterivirus* family. Infections range from acute, clinical infection to the more common subclinical infection and are largely dependent on a variety of factors including strain, genetics, immunocompetency, breed susceptibility and route of infection. Outbreaks of EVA have been reported. Transmission occurs primarily via respiratory (aerosolization of secretions) or venereal routes (breeding to an acute or chronically infected stallion). Clinical signs of acute infections include fever, respiratory signs, edema at various sites (ie, supraorbital, limb, preputial, etc.), depression, petechial hemorrhages, and conjunctivitis, to name a few. Regarding natural infections, mortality is more common in foals that develop severe interstitial pneumonia or aborted fetuses.[22–24]

Maintenance and transmission of EAV in the equine population is a multilayered process. Acutely infected horses can shed via aerosolization of respiratory particles as well as other secretions (ie, urine). Horizontal transmission occurs when there is direct/close contact between an infected and naïve animal. Nasal shedding can persist for 7 to 14 days during the acute phase. Venereal transmission occurs when a mare is exposed to semen from an acutely infected or carrier stallion during natural cover or artificial insemination.[23,25] Acutely infected mares shed virus via the respiratory route, thereby being a critical player in the development of an outbreak if in close proximity to susceptible horses. In addition, donor mares exposed to EAV-infected semen can transmit the virus to embryo recipient mares.[26] Transplacental transmission can result in congenital infection with the foal developing severe interstitial pneumonia.[27-29] Finally contaminated instruments, phantoms, clothing, etc. act as fomites for transmission as well.[30-32] The carrier stallion is critical to maintenance of the virus in the equine population. Approximately 10% to 70% of stallions will become persistently infected with the carrier state lasting anywhere from weeks to years to even a lifetime. EAV genetic variation appears to occur within the reproductive tract of the carrier stallion leading to the development of novel variants.[23,25,33-36]

EVA is a well-known cause of abortion in the equine population and can produce outbreak situations[23,37,38] Abortion can occur without pre-existing signs anywhere from 2 to 10 months of gestation.[23,24] One study exposed a group of 14 pregnant mares to known infected mares with EAV. All mares in the study become seropositive after exposure to the virus. Virus was isolated from the nasopharynx in 35% of the pregnant mares. Following exposure, 10 of the pregnant mares aborted approximately 1 to 2 months afterward. Of that group, virus was isolated in the tissues (placenta, spleen, lung, and kidney) of eight of the aborted fetuses. Placenta was the most common tissue from which virus was isolated.[39] Reported microscopic lesions in fetuses aborted due to EVA infection can vary from none to inflammation and necrosis of the placenta, brain, lymphoid tissues (spleen, thymus, lymph nodes), and liver frequently accompanied by vasculitis. When present, lesions in the placenta tend to be the most severe.[24,38] Vasculitis is expected as the virus is known to target blood vessels. Confirmation of abortion due to EVA can be achieved via virus isolation, IHC or PCR of fetal tissues.[23] Suggested tissues for testing include placenta, lung, spleen, lymphoid tissue, and fetal fluids.[22]

Vaccination guidelines for seronegative mares to be bred to carrier stallions include vaccination with the modified live vaccine 3 weeks or more before breeding or post-foaling with annual boosters thereafter. After vaccination, the mare should be isolated for 21 days. If the mare is seropositive then breeding to an EAV stallion can occur without vaccination. Following breeding, these mares should be isolated for 24 hours. Vaccination of pregnant mares during the last 2 months of gestation can result in abortion.[22,23,40]

Equine infectious anemia
Equine infectious anemia (EIA) is a lentivirus transmitted via bloodsucking insects (ie, horsefly) or iatrogenically through contaminated blood products or instruments. Infection can result in an acute, subacute, or chronic stage. Clinical signs associated with the acute stage include pronounced pyrexia, thrombocytopenia, anemia, and swelling of the ventral abdomen and limbs. The subacute to chronic scenarios manifest as intermittent fever, anemia, weight loss, swelling, and splenomegaly. Although in some cases, the horse may have an inapparent infection. In general, severity of clinical signs is often based on the viral strain.[41,42]

Pregnant mares with EIA can result in abortion or birth of foals that may or may not be seropositive. Possible routes of transmission from mare to fetus/foal include transplacental, via colostrum/milk or vectors. In an experimental setting, pony mares (agar gel immunodiffusion [AGID] negative for EIA) were bred to stallions and the resultant pregnancies were confirmed. Fetuses inoculated with a cell-adapted Wyoming strain of EIA at or before 203 days resulted in resorption or abortion with two fetuses testing positive for EIA. Fetuses infected 204 days and after resulted in a live birth. The live foals that were seropositive at birth died within the first 60 days of life.[43] Given the development of the immune response during gestation, it was suggested that the ability of the fetus to mount an immune response was an important determinant to the outcome of resorption/abortion versus carrying to term and resulting in a live birth.[43] Another study followed the outcome of foals born to 52 broodmares seropositive for EIA. Of the progeny, 12 of the 52 foals were positive at birth. Five of the foals were produced from mares that showed clinical signs of EIA during gestation. The remaining 7 foals were born to seropositive mares who did not show clinical signs. One mare was aborted at 8 months gestation with the fetus testing positive.[44] In another study, foals born to carrier mares underwent serial testing for EIA. Ninety percent of the foals who initially testing seropositive were found to be seronegative between approximately 2 to 6 months of age.[45] Another study also supported the finding that foals nursing seropositive dams can eventually convert to EIA negative status on the AGID test.[46] In summary, broodmares who show clinical signs of EIA during gestation are more of a concern for abortion depending on the stage of gestation.

AGID and ELISA tests are available for diagnosis of EIA in the horse population. These test modalities have been found to perform with good concordance.[47] In the literature, fetal testing has relied on AGID testing of blood or inoculation of other animals with fetal tissue. Control of EIA is multifactorial, including euthanasia or lifelong quarantine of positive animals, disinfection of various instruments after each use, prohibited repeated use of needles and syringes on multiple animals, fly control and up-to-date Coggins testing to confirm a negative EIA result for interstate travel.[41]

Bacterial Diseases

Leptospirosis

Leptospiral abortion is caused by a spiral bacterium that infects humans and animals. Greater than 10 species and 300 serotypes have been recognized. *Leptospira interrogans* serovar Pomona (type Kennewicki) is the most common serovar (incidental and pathogenic) for horses in North America and *Leptospira kirschneri* serovar grippotyphosa has been documented less frequently.[48,49] The wildlife reservoirs include opossums, striped skunks, racoons, and foxes. Exposure of horses occurs through direct contact with infected urine, contaminated water sources or reproductive tissues and fluids. Infection of pregnant mares with leptospirosis can cause abortion, stillbirth and/or placentitis. The incidence of leptospiral abortion is variable between years with variation in rainfall and flooding possibly influencing exposure rates.

In most abortions caused by leptospires, the organism can easily be detected in fetal and maternal tissues. Abortion typically occurs approximately 2 to 4 weeks after infection, often late in gestation without premonitory signs. A substantial number of mares that are infected will not abort. Occasionally a small, weak, live foal will be produced with some foals displaying icterus. Mares may shed leptospires in the urine for up 14 weeks. In a pathologic description of 71 cases of leptospiral abortion/still birth, 80% of cases had gross lesions observed. Changes in the placenta are variable, ranging from normal in appearance to large areas of edema and necrosis of the chorion. Funisitis (inflammation of the umbilical cord) and cystic adenomatous allantoic hyperplasia, whereas not specific to leptospiral abortion, are often observed. Microscopically, inflammation, necrosis, and vasculitis may be observed.[50] The fetus often has a grossly enlarged liver and kidneys, both with areas of necrosis and hemorrhage. The classic renal lesion is radiating white streaks (**Fig. 3**). The fetus may be icteric. The most common microscopic lesions are a suppurative tubular nephritis

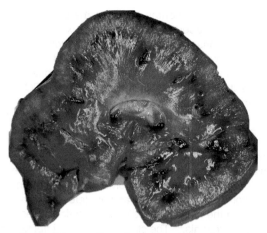

Fig. 3. Kidney from a fetus with a confirmed abortion due to leptospirosis. Radiating linear white streaks are scattered throughout the cortex.

and hepatocellular disassociation with hepatitis and hepatopathy with giant cells. Additional lesions may be observed in the heart, lung, brain and lymphoid organs.[50,51] Diagnosis can be based on fluorescent antibody testing, PCR for leptospires on the fetal kidney, or microscopic findings. In addition, the microscopic agglutination test can be performed on fetal heart blood.[48] Following identification of a leptospiral abortion the mare should ideally be isolated for several weeks. It is unclear if antimicrobial treatment following abortion decreases the period of bacterial shedding. Prevention includes decreasing exposure to contaminated water sources, wildlife vectors, and appropriate isolation protocols. Vaccination of mares at risk for exposure to *L interrogans* serovar Pomona (type Kennewicki) is recommended as proper vaccination is expected to prevent bacteremia.[48] In addition, paired serum titers in pregnant mares may help predict exposure and risk.[52]

Potomac horse fever

Potomac horse fever (PHF) is caused by the Gram-negative obligate bacterium *Neorickettsia risticii* (formerly *Ehrlichia risticii*). The disease was first recognized in 1979 in the Potomac River region and has since been reported in Canada, South America, Europe and various portions of the United States[53–55] In addition, a novel species, *N findlayensis*, has been found to cause PHF in horses.[56,57] Common clinical signs of PHF include diarrhea, fever, anorexia, laminitis, and abortion. In one retrospective, the most common presentation was diarrhea followed by fever.[58] Regarding pathogenesis, the bacteria infect trematodes that then parasitize water snails.[59–63] The snails release infected cercariae that progress to metacercariae in the second intermediate host, aquatic insects. Reported infected aquatic insects that act as a vector include mayflies, caddis flies, and dragon flies to name a few.[64–66] Horses are infected by either ingesting the infected trematodes or infected intermediate hosts. Clinical cases are most common in the summer months. Horses grazing near water sources have potential increased exposure to aquatic insects harboring the infected trematodes or the trematodes themselves.

There are multiple reports of PHF causing abortion in experimental and natural infection.[67–70] In experimental infections, abortion occurred anywhere from 65 to 111 days post-inoculation.[67,68] In one experimental model, the organism was detected in the fetal tissues 4 months after the mare was infected.[69] In a report describing natural infection, abortion occurred approximately 80 days after clinical signs.[71] Reported fetal lesions on postmortem examination include lymphohistiocytic enterocolitis, hepatitis, myocarditis, lymphadenitis, and lymphoid hyperplasia or depletion in various lymphoid tissues. The placenta is grossly and microscopically normal in natural infection. Detection of the organism via PCR or cell culture has been reported in lymph node, thymus, liver, colon, spleen and bone marrow.[70,71] PHF is a worthwhile consideration for pregnant mares diagnosed with PHF as abortion can occur months after infection.

Ascending placentitis

Ascending placentitis refers to bacterial or fungal infection of the chorioallantois via the cervix. This may occur with cervical incompetency or softening during vaginitis, pneumovagina or secondary ovulations. Anatomic defects of the caudal reproductive tract are often present in the mare. Ascending placentitis causes abortion, premature birth, and delivery of septic foals.[52] The classical signs of infection include premature udder development and vaginal discharge; however, many mares will not show these signs.[52,72] High value and high-risk mares may be evaluated from the 7th month of gestation for evidence of placentitis using a combination of physical examination, endocrinological and ultrasonographic parameters.[52] Common treatment includes antibiotics, non-steroidal anti-inflammatories, pentoxifylline and altrenogest or progesterone. The most common bacteria isolated is *Streptococcus sp.* with other common bacteria including *E coli, Pseudomonas, Klebsiella* and *S sp.* The gross and microscopic appearance is similar with all bacteria. The chorionic surface is discolored brown to tan with variable exudate, most severe at the cervical star and often extending toward the placental body (**Fig. 4**). Fetal fluids may be discolored or cloudy.[73] Fetal lesions depend on the degree of fetal bacteremia or septicemia and range from none to areas of inflammation and necrosis throughout multiple organs. Fungal infections subjectively have a thicker, more "leather like" appearance with *Aspergillus sp.* being the most isolated fungus.[74] Diagnosis following parturition or abortion is made with examination of the chorioallantois and culture of the affected areas. The common organisms isolated in cases of ascending placentitis are those found in the vaginal microflora and so correlation of gross or microscopic evidence of placentitis is recommended to confirm the significance of positive culture results.[73]

Nocardioform placentitis

Nocardioform placentitis is associated with gram-positive branching actinomycetes of which *Crossiella equi* and *Amycolatopsis sp.* are the most common. These

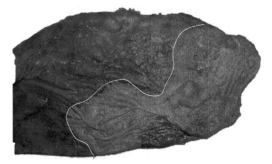

Fig. 4. Chronic ascending bacterial placentitis. A locally extensive well demarcated tan focus begins at the cervical star and extends to the body (white line).

actinomycetes are soil organisms, and the pathogenesis of infection remains unknown.[75] Attempts to reproduce clinical placentitis with inoculation via the bloodstream, transcervical or orally have failed.[76] A strong association with weather patterns has been identified with a higher incidence of nocardioform placentitis in foaling seasons associated with hot, dry periods in August and September. Cases have been reported in multiple regions of the United States and world.[75,77–79] Mares may show no clinical signs or may have premature mammary gland development. Transrectal ultrasound may have a normal combined thickness of the uteroplacental unit and transcutaneous abdominal ultrasound may be required to see abnormalities.

Pregnancy outcomes include abortion, birth of small underweight and premature foals, or birth of normal foals. The placenta will classically have accumulation of several thick, brown-tan mucoid material on the chorionic surface, most often at the bifurcation of the placental horns. This appearance classifies nocardioform placentitis as one of the common causes of mucoid placentitis. Although the predilection site is the bifurcation of the horns, lesions can be seen in any site of the chorion.[75] Grossly, the lesions of nocardioform placentitis range from thickened, tan, and irregular chorion to thin, avillous areas and the amount of mucoid material is highly variable with a portion of cases only having this material observed microscopically. The bacteria are most often visualized at the edge of the lesion, and this is the preferred sampling site for culture, histopathology and molecular testing (**Fig. 5**). PCR is available for C equi, Amycolatopsis sp and S sp.[80] All have been identified in normal placental tissue and the latter is also considered a potential environmental contaminant and so test results should be interpreted in the context of the clinical appearance of the placenta.[75] To date, there is no known prevention as the pathogenesis is unknown. Regular evaluation of the fetal placental unit, identification of mares with premature udder development and implementation of appropriate antimicrobial therapy and supportive care will help a portion of these mares produce a live foal.

Rhodoccocus equi

Sporadic cases of placentitis and abortion due to Rhodococcus equi have been reported. Abortion has been identified in mid-to late-term fetuses. Inflammation with a predominance of macrophages was observed within the fetal lungs and placenta. The authors suspected a hematogenous route on infection based on the distribution throughout the allantois. Pure culture of R equi from the placenta, liver, kidney, fetal stomach fluid and lungs confirmed the diagnosis as well as visualization of Gram-positive coccobacilli within macrophages.[81–83]

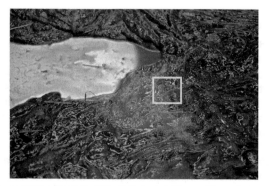

Fig. 5. Mucoid placentitis caused by Crossiella equi. The preferred sampling site is at the edge of the area of avillous chorion where there are raised, red and tan foci (white box).

Salmonella abortus equi

Salmonella enterica subspecies enterica serovar abortus equi (S abortus equi) is a recognized cause of abortion in both horses and donkeys.[84] Abortion induced by this pathogen causes loss in late pregnancy and neonatal sepsis.[85] The organism continues to be of concern in Asian and African countries where cases are reported commonly. In Europe, the United States, and Argentina, sporadic cases are reported.[84–86] The bacteria are transmitted through consumption of food sources contaminated with vaginal secretions from aborting animals. Severe disease outbreaks have been described with high foal mortality. Diagnosis is by culture of the bacteria from fetal tissues. Horses infected with S abortus equi may become long-term carries and continue to contaminate the environment.

Mare Reproductive Loss Syndrome

In the spring of 2001 an outbreak of early fetal loss (EFL), late-term abortions, stillbirths and neonatal foal deaths occurred in central Kentucky. In addition, cases of pericarditis and unilateral uveitis were reported. Most losses occurred in April and May. The combination of fetal losses was termed "mare reproductive loss syndrome" (MRLS). An estimated 3500 foals were lost to MRLS in 2001 with cases reported in multiple states outside of KY.[87,88]

Cases of EFL were typically detected during fetal sexing with an absent or slow fetal heartbeat and increased echogenicity of fetal fluids. In some cases, vulvar discharge, fever and colic were observed in the mare. Postmortem findings typically seen in cases of MRLS include fetuses in good postmortem condition of appropriate gestational weight and size. Hemorrhage was present in the lungs of some fetuses and the allantochorion. The amniotic segment of the umbilical cord is typically enlarged, edematous with gray-yellow discoloration. Neutrophilic pneumonia and neutrophilic and histiocytic funisitis are the typical microscopic findings. The most commonly isolated bacteria are Streptococcus and Actinobacillus spp.[88] Analysis of risk factors indicates that exposure to the eastern tent caterpillar (ETC), Malacosoma americanum, presence of cherry trees and stocking density increased the risk of MRLS. The ability of the ETC to produce abortion experimentally was confirmed although the exact syndrome of MRLS was not reproduced[88–90] There is continued interest in understanding the exact pathogenesis of MRLS.[91] At this time in central KY the syndrome is seen very sporadically in individual abortions with environmental management on farms to reduce exposure to the ETC appearing successful.[92] In Australia equine amnionitis and fetal loss have also been linked to caterpillar exposure.[93]

Uncommon or Uncertain Causes of Infectious Abortion

In a study focused on detection of uncommon causes of equine abortion, the authors used real-time PCR to detect DNA of Neospora caninum, Coxiella burnettii, and Chlamydophila abortus. These were found in three, six and one case, respectively, out of 407 cases of abortion. In no case in this study were these pathogens confirmed as the primary cause of abortion.[94] Neospora caninum has been detected in fetal tissues and in congenitally infected foals, confirming transplacental infection. These animals lack histologic evidence of tissue changes, and so N caninum as a cause of abortion could be confirmed.[95]

Chlamydia psittaci can cause abortion with reports from Germany, Hungary and Australia.[96] The importance of C psittaci in equine reproductive losses is currently being investigated and warrants concern due to the zoonotic potential of this disease, particularly in cases where humans are exposed to an aborted fetus and fetal fluids.

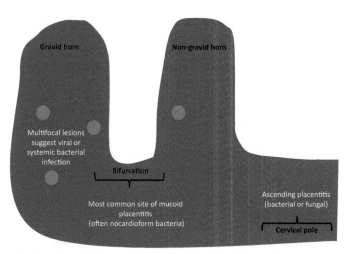

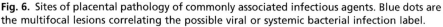

Fig. 6. Sites of placental pathology of commonly associated infectious agents. Blue dots are the multifocal lesions correlating the possible viral or systemic bacterial infection label.

The prevalence of *C psittaci* in cases of equine abortion in Australia has been investigated with a range in prevalence from 6.5% to 21.1%.[96]

Encephalitozoon cuniculi is a microsporidian organism that infects mammals and some avian species. Sporadic cases of equine abortion have been reported. Placentitis and abortion have been observed with lesions in the horns of the placenta. Interstitial nephritis, placentitis and synovitis have been described. Diagnosis is via molecular or ultrastructural detection of the organism.[97,98]

SUMMARY

A variety of infectious agents including viral, bacterial, and fungal organisms can cause equine abortion and placentitis. Knowledge of normal anatomy and the common pattern distribution of different infectious agents (**Fig. 6**) will assist the practitioner in evaluating the fetus and/or placenta, collecting appropriate samples for further testing, and in some cases, forming a presumptive diagnosis. In all cases, it is recommended to confirm the diagnosis with molecular, serologic or microbiological testing. If a causative agent can be identified, then appropriate biosecurity and vaccination measures can be instituted on the farm. Importantly, many cases of abortion will not have an infectious etiology, but the exclusion of infectious diseases is an important part of all cases of fetal loss.

DISCLOSURE

The authors have nothing to disclose.

REFERENCES

1. Slater J. Equine Herpesviruses. In: Maureen T, editor. Sellon DCL. Equine infectious diseases, 151, 2nd edition. St. Louis: Saunders Elsevier; 2014. p. 138.

2. Allen G. Epidemic disease caused by Equine herpesvirus-1: recommendations for prevention and control. Equine Vet Education 2002;14:136–42.

3. Slater J, Borchers K, Thackray A, et al. The trigeminal ganglion is a location for equine herpesvirus 1 latency and reactivation in the horse. J Gen Virol 1994; 75:2007–16.

4. Edington N, Bridges C, Huckle A. Experimental reactivation of equid herpesvirus 1 (EHV 1) following the administration of corticosteroids. Equine Vet J 1985;17: 369–72.

5. Edington N, Smyth B, Griffiths L. The role of endothelial cell infection in the endometrium, placenta and foetus of equid herpesvirus 1 (EHV-1) abortions. J Comp Pathol 1991;104:379–87.

6. Smith KC, Mumford JA, Lakhani K. A comparison of equid herpesvirus-1 (EHV-1) vascular lesions in the early versus late pregnant equine uterus. J Comp Pathol 1996;114(3):231–47.

7. Smith K, Mumford J, Lakhani K. A comparison of equid herpesvirus-1 (EHV-1) vascular lesions in the early versus late pregnant equine uterus. J Comp Pathol 1996;114:231–47.

8. Smith K, Whitwell KE, Binns M, et al. Abortion of virologically negative foetuses following experimental challenge of pregnant pony mares with equid herpesvirus 1. Equine Vet J 1992;24:256–9.

9. Gardiner DW, Lunn DP, Goehring LS, et al. Strain impact on equine herpesvirus type 1 (EHV-1) abortion models: Viral loads in fetal and placental tissues and foals. Vaccine 2012;30:6564–72.

10. Garvey M, Lyons R, Hector RD, et al. Molecular characterisation of equine herpesvirus 1 isolates from cases of abortion, respiratory and neurological disease in Ireland between 1990 and 2017. Pathogens 2019;8:7.

11. Allen G, Yeargan M, Turtinen L, et al. A new field strain of equine abortion virus (equine herpesvirus-1) among Kentucky horses. Am J Vet Res 1985;46:138–40.

12. Damiani AM, de Vries M, Reimers G, et al. A severe equine herpesvirus type 1 (EHV-1) abortion outbreak caused by a neuropathogenic strain at a breeding farm in northern Germany. Vet Microbiol 2014;172:555–62.

13. Stasiak K, Rola J, Ploszay G, et al. Detection of the neuropathogenic variant of equine herpesvirus 1 associated with abortions in mares in Poland. BMC Vet Res 2015;11:102.

14. Reed SM, Toribio RE. Equine herpesvirus 1 and 4. Vet Clin Equine Pract 2004;20: 631–42.

15. Schlafer DH. Equid herpesvirus 1 abortion in horses In: Maxie MG. In: Jubb Kennedy, Palmar's, editors. Pathology of domestic animals. 6th ed. St. Louis: Elsevier; 2016. p. 435–7.

16. Ballagi-Pordany A, Klingeborn B, Flensburg J, et al. Equine herpesvirus type 1: detection of viral DNA sequences in aborted fetuses with the polymerase chain reaction. Vet Microbiol 1990;22:373–81.

17. Lunn DP, Davis-Poynter N, Flaminio MJBF, et al. Equine Herpesvirus-1 Consensus Statement. J Vet Intern Med 2009;23:450–61.

18. Mumford JA, Rossdale PD, Jessett DM, et al. Serological and virological investigations of an equid herpesvirus 1 (EHV-1) abortion storm on a stud farm in 1985. J Reprod Fertil Suppl 1987;35:509–18.

19. Bürki F, Rossmanith W, Nowotny N, et al. Viraemia and abortions are not prevented by two commercial Equine Herpesvirus-1 vaccines after experimental challenge of horses. Vet Q 1990;12:80–6.

20. Bryans J, Allen G. Application of a chemically inactivated, adjuvanted vaccine to control abortigenic infection of mares by equine herpesvirus I. Dev Biol standardization 1982;52:493–8.

21. Burrows R, Goodridge D, Denyer M. Trials of an inactivated equid herpesvirus 1 vaccine: challenge with a subtype 1 virus. The Vet Rec 1984;114:369–74.
22. Balasuriya UB. Equine viral arteritis. Vet Clin Equine Pract 2014;30:543–60.
23. Balasuriya U, Carossino M, Timoney P. Equine viral arteritis: a respiratory and reproductive disease of significant economic importance to the equine industry. Equine Vet Education 2018;30:497–512.
24. Del Piero F. Equine viral arteritis. Vet Pathol 2000;37:287–96.
25. Timoney P, McCollum W, Murphy T, et al. The carrier state in equine arteritis virus infection in the stallion with specific emphasis on the venereal mode of virus transmission. J Reprod Fertil Suppl 1987;35:95–102.
26. Broaddus C, Balasuriya U, Timoney P, et al. Infection of embryos following insemination of donor mares with equine arteritis virus infective semen. Theriogenology 2011;76:47–60.
27. Golnik W, Michalska Z, Michalak T. Natural equine viral arteritis in foals. Schweizer Archiv fur Tierheilkunde 1981;123:523–33.
28. VAALA WE, Hamir A, Dubovi E, et al. Fatal, congenitally acquired infection with equine arteritis virus in a neonatal thoroughbred. Equine Vet J 1992;24:155–8.
29. Del Piero F, Wilkins PA, Lopez J, et al. Equine viral arteritis in newborn foals: clinical, pathological, serological, microbiological and immunohistochemical observations. Equine Vet J 1997;29:178–85.
30. Timoney PJ, McCollum WH. Equine viral arteritis. Vet Clin North America: Equine Pract 1993;9:295–309.
31. Timoney P, McCollum W. Equine viral arteritis—epidemiology and control. J Equine Vet Sci 1988;8:54–9.
32. Guthrie A, Howell P, Hedges J, et al. Lateral transmission of equine arteritis virus among Lipizzaner stallions in South Africa. Equine Vet J 2003;35:596–600.
33. Balasuriya UB, Hedges JF, Nadler SA, et al. Genetic stability of equine arteritis virus during horizontal and vertical transmission in an outbreak of equine viral arteritis. J Gen Virol 1999;80:1949–58.
34. Balasuriya UR, Hedges J, Maclachlan NJ. Molecular epidemiology and evolution of equine arteritis virus. Boston, MA: The Nidoviruses: Springer; 2001. p. 19–24.
35. Balasuriya UB, Hedges JF, Smalley VL, et al. Genetic characterization of equine arteritis virus during persistent infection of stallions. J Gen Virol 2004;85:379–90.
36. Hedges JF, Balasuriya UB, Timoney PJ, et al. Genetic divergence with emergence of novel phenotypic variants of equine arteritis virus during persistent infection of stallions. J Virol 1999;73:3672–81.
37. van der Meulen K, Caij A, Nauwynck H, et al. An outbreak of equine viral arteritis abortion in Belgium. Vlaams Diergeneeskundig Tijdschrift 2001;70:221–2.
38. Johnson B, Baldwin C, Timoney P, et al. Arteritis in equine fetuses aborted due to equine viral arteritis. Vet Pathol 1991;28:248–50.
39. Cole JR, Hall RF, Gosser HS, et al. Transmissibility and abortogenic effect of equine viral arteritis in mares. J Am Vet Med Assoc 1986;189:769–71.
40. Broaddus CC, Balasuriya UB, White JL, et al. Evaluation of the safety of vaccinating mares against equine viral arteritis during mid or late gestation or during the immediate postpartum period. J Am Vet Med Assoc 2011;238:741–50.
41. Sellon DC. Equine infectious anemia. Vet Clin North America: Equine Pract 1993;9:321–36.
42. Sellon DC, Fuller FJ, McGuire TC. The immunopathogenesis of equine infectious anemia virus. Virus Res 1994;32:111–38.
43. Issel CJ, Cook RF, Adams WV. Foetal responses to experimental infection with a cell-adapted strain of equine infectious anemia virus. In: Plowright W, Rossdale PD,

Wade JF, editors. Equine Infectious Diseases VI. Proceedings of the Sixth International Conference. Newmarket: R&W Publications; 1992. p. 249.

44. Kemen M, Coggins L. Equine infectious anemia: transmission from infected mares to foals. J Am Vet Med Assoc 1972;161:496–9.

45. Burns S. Equine infectious anemia: plasma clearance times of passively transferred antibody in foals. J Am Vet Med Assoc 1974;164(1):64–5.

46. Tashjian R. Transmission and clinical evaluation of an equine infectious anemia herd and their offspring over a 13-year period. J Am Vet Med Assoc 1984;184: 282–8.

47. Issel CJ, Rwambo PM, Montelaro RC. Evolution of equine infectious anemia diagnostic tests: recognition of a need for detection of anti-EIAV glycoprotein antibodies. InEquine Infectious Diseases V. Proceedings of the Fifth International Conference. University Press of Kentucky; 1988. p. 196–200.

48. Divers TJ, Chang YF, Irby NL, et al. Leptospirosis: An important infectious disease in North American horses. Equine Vet J 2019;51:287–92.

49. Timoney JF, Kalimuthusamy N, Velineni S, et al. A unique genotype of Leptospira interrogans serovar Pomona type kennewicki is associated with equine abortion. Vet Microbiol 2011;150:349–53.

50. Poonacha KB, Donahue JM, Giles RC, et al. Leptospirosis in equine fetuses, stillborn foals, and placentas. Vet Pathol 1993;30:362–9.

51. Ellis WA, Bryson DG, Obrien JJ, et al. Leptospiral infection in aborted equine fetuses. Equine Vet J 1983;15:321–4.

52. LeBlanc MM. Ascending Placentitis in the Mare: An Update. Reprod Domest Anim 2010;45:28–34.

53. Holland CJ, Ristic M, Cole AI, et al. Isolation, experimental transmission, and characterization of causative agent of Potomac horse fever. Science 1985;227: 522–4.

54. Madigan JE, Pusterla N. Ehrlichial diseases. Vet Clin North America: Equine Pract 2000;16:487–99.

55. Knowles R, Anderson C, Shipley W, et al. Acute equine diarrhea syndrome (AEDS): a preliminary report. Am Assoc Equine Pract Annu Convention 1983;353–7.

56. Teymournejad O, Lin M, Bekebrede H, et al. Isolation and Molecular Analysis of a Novel Neorickettsia Species That Causes Potomac Horse Fever. mBio 2020;11: e03429.

57. Budachetri K, Lin M, Yan Q, et al. Real-Time PCR differential detection of neorickettsia findlayensis and N. risticii in cases of potomac horse fever. J Clin Microbiol 2022;60(7). e00250-00222.

58. Bertin F, Reising A, Slovis N, et al. Clinical and clinicopathological factors associated with survival in 44 horses with equine neorickettsiosis (Potomac horse Fever). J Vet Intern Med 2013;27:1528–34.

59. Pusterla N, Leutenegger C, Sigrist B, et al. Detection and quantitation of Ehrlichia risticii genomic DNA in infected horses and snails by real-time PCR. Vet Parasitol 2000;90:129–35.

60. Pusterla N, Madigan JE, Chae J-S, et al. Helminthic transmission and isolation of Ehrlichia risticii, the causative agent of Potomac horse fever, by using trematode stages from freshwater stream snails. J Clin Microbiol 2000;38:1293–7.

61. Madigan JE, Chae J-s, Pusterla N. Potomac horse fever: identification and transmission of the causative agent via trematodes of freshwater snails. Lexington: American Association of Equine Practitioners (AAEP); 1999.

62. Madigan J, Pusterla N. Life cycle of Potomac Horse Fever - implications for diagnosis, treatment, and control: a review. Lexington: American Association of Equine Practitioners (AAEP); 2005.
63. Barlough JE, Reubel GH, Madigan JE, et al. Detection of Ehrlichia risticii, the agent of Potomac horse fever, in freshwater stream snails (Pleuroceridae: Juga spp.) from northern California. Appl Environ Microbiol 1998;64:2888–93.
64. Chae J-s, Pusterla N, Johnson E, et al. Infection of aquatic insects with trematode metacercariae carrying Ehrlichia risticii, the cause of Potomac horse fever. J Med Entomol 2000;37:619–25.
65. Mott J, Muramatsu Y, Seaton E, et al. Molecular analysis of Neorickettsia risticii in adult aquatic insects in Pennsylvania, in horses infected by ingestion of insects, and isolated in cell culture. J Clin Microbiol 2002;40:690–3.
66. Wilson JH, Pusterla N, Bengfort JM, et al. Incrimination of mayflies as a vector of Potomac Horse Fever in an outbreak in Minnesota. Med AAEP Proc 2006;52: 324–8.
67. Long M, Goetz T, Kakoma I, et al. Evaluation of fetal infection and abortion in pregnant ponies experimentally infected with Ehrlichia risticii. Am J Vet Res 1995;56:1307–16.
68. Long M, Goetz T, Kakoma I, et al. Isolation of Ehrlichia risticii from the aborted fetus of an infected mare. Vet Rec 1992;131(16):370.
69. Dawson J, Ristic M, Holland C, et al. Isolation of Ehrlichia risticii, the causative agent of Potomac horse fever, from the fetus of an experimentally infected mare. The Vet Rec 1987;121:232.
70. Coffman EA, Abd-Eldaim M, Craig LE. Abortion in a horse following Neorickettsia risticii infection. J Vet Diagn Invest 2008;20:827–30.
71. Long M, Goetz T, Whiteley H, et al. Identification of Ehrlichia risticii as the causative agent of two equine abortions following natural maternal infection. J Vet Diagn Invest 1995;7:201–5.
72. Govaere J, Roels K, Ververs C, et al. Ascending placentitis in the mare. Vlaams Diergeneeskundig Tijdschrift 2018;87:115–26.
73. Cummins C, Carrington S, Fitzpatrick E, et al. Ascending placentitis in the mare: A review. Irish Vet J 2008;61:307–13.
74. Hong CB, Donahue JM, Giles RC, et al. Etiology and Pathology of Equine Placentitis. J Vet Diagn Invest 1993;5:56–63.
75. Fedorka CE, Scoggin KE, Ruby RE, et al. Clinical, pathologic, and epidemiologic features of nocardioform placentitis in the mare. Theriogenology 2021;171: 155–61.
76. Canisso IF, Ball BA, Erol E, et al. Attempts to induce nocardioform placentitis (Crossiela equi) experimentally in mares. Equine Vet J 2015;47:91–5.
77. Cattoli G, Vascellari M, Corro M, et al. First case of equine nocardioform placentitis caused by Crossiella equi in Europe. Vet Rec 2004;154:730–1.
78. Christensen BW, Roberts JF, Pozor MA, et al. Nocardioform placentitis with isolation of Amycolatopsis spp in a Florida-bred mare. Javma-Journal Am Vet Med Assoc 2006;228:1234–9.
79. Volkmann DH, Williams JH, Henton MM, et al. The first reported case of equine nocardioform placentitis in South Africa. J South Afr Vet Assoc 2001;72:235–8.
80. Erol E, Sells SF, Williams NM, et al. An investigation of a recent outbreak of nocardioform placentitis caused abortions in horses. Vet Microbiol 2012;158:425–30.
81. Patterson-Kane JC, Donahue JM, Harrison LR. Placentitis, fetal pneumonia, and abortion due to Rhodococcus equi infection in a Thoroughbred. J Vet Diagn Invest 2002;14:157–9.

82. Szeredi L, Molnar T, Glavits R, et al. Two cases of equine abortion caused by Rhodococcus equi. Vet Pathol 2006;43:208–11.
83. Nakamura Y, Nishi H, Katayama Y, et al. Abortion in a thoroughbred mare associated with an infection with avirulent Rhodococcus equi. Vet Rec 2007;161: 342–6.
84. Wang H, Liu KJ, Sun YH, et al. Abortion in donkeys associated with Salmonella abortus equi infection. Equine Vet J 2019;51:756–9.
85. Grandolfo E, Parisi A, Ricci A, et al. High mortality in foals associated with Salmonella enterica subsp enterica Abortusequi infection in Italy. J Vet Diagn Invest 2018;30:483–5.
86. Stazi M, Pellegrini M, Rampacci E, et al. A new Montanide (TM) Seppic IMS1313-adjuvanted autogenous vaccine as a useful emergency tool to resolve a Salmonella enterica subsp. enterica serovar abortus equi abortion outbreak in mares. Open Vet J 2022;12:303–7.
87. Sebastian M, Gantz MG, Tobin T, et al. The mare reproductive loss syndrome and the eastern tent caterpillar: a toxicokinetic/statistical analysis with clinical, epidemiologic, and mechanistic implications. Vet Ther 2003;4:324–39.
88. Sebastian MM, Bernard WV, Riddle TW, et al. REVIEW paper: mare reproductive loss syndrome. Vet Pathol 2008;45:710–22.
89. Webb BA, Barney WE, Dahlman DL, et al. Eastern tent caterpillars (Malacosoma americanum) cause mare reproductive loss syndrome. J Insect Physiol 2004;50: 185–93.
90. Potter DA, Foss L, Baumler RE, et al. Managing Eastern tent caterpillars Malacosoma americanum (F) on horse farms to reduce risk of mare reproductive loss syndrome. Pest Manag Sci 2005;61:3–15.
91. Swerczek TW. An alternative model for fetal loss disorders associated with mare reproductive loss syndrome. Anim Nutr 2020;6:217–24.
92. Bernard WV, LeBlanc MM, Webb BA, et al. Evaluation of early fetal loss induced by gavage with eastern tent caterpillars in pregnant mares. J Am Vet Med Assoc 2004;225:717–21.
93. Cawdell-Smith AJ, Todhunter KH, Anderson ST, et al. Equine amnionitis and fetal loss: mare abortion following experimental exposure to Processionary caterpillars (Ochrogaster lunifer). Equine Vet J 2012;44:282–8.
94. Leon A, Richard E, Fortier C, et al. Molecular detection of Coxiella burnetii and Neospora caninum in equine aborted foetuses and neonates. Prev Vet Med 2012;104:179–83.
95. Veronesi F, Diaferia M, Mandara MT, et al. Neospora spp. infection associated with equine abortion and/or stillbirth rate. Vet Res Commun 2008;32:S223–6.
96. Akter R, Sansom FM, El-Hage CM, et al. A 25-year retrospective study of Chlamydia psittaci in association with equine reproductive loss in Australia. J Med Microbiol 2021;70(2):001284.
97. Patterson-Kane JC, Caplazi P, Rurangirwa F, et al. Encephalitozoon cuniculi placentitis and abortion in a Quarterhorse mare. J Vet Diagn Invest 2003;15:57–9.
98. Vanrensburg IBJ, Volkmann DH, Soley JT, et al. Encephalitozoon Infection in a Still-Born Foal. J South Afr Vet Association-Tydskrif Van Die Suid-Afrikaanse Veterinere Vereniging 1991;62:130–2.

Hendra Virus
An Update on Diagnosis, Vaccination, and Biosecurity Protocols for Horses

Xueli Wang, DVM, Jessica C. Wise, BVetBio/BVSc, MANZCVS, DVStud, DipECEIM, Allison J. Stewart, BVSc (Hons I), MS, DACVIM, DACVECC, PhD, MANZCVS*

KEYWORDS

- Zoonotic • Emerging zoonosis • Infectious disease • Respiratory • Neurology
- One health

KEY POINTS

- Hendra virus (HeV) is an Australian zoonotic disease with a high mortality rate in horses and humans.
- Nonspecific clinical signs such as fever, anorexia and depression are the most common initial clinical signs, while neurological and respiratory symptoms are the most common terminal signs in horses infected with HeV.
- Equivac HeV is an effective and safe commercial vaccine for horses against HeV and the main strategy to secondarily protect humans.
- It is critical for individual veterinarians and veterinary clinics to implement protocols to avoid human exposure by minimizing the possibility of disease transmission and by identifying infected horses.

INTRODUCTION

Hendra virus (HeV) belongs to the family Paramyxoviridae, under the genus Henipavirus (named after Hendra and Nipah viruses).[1] Paramyxoviruses are large, enveloped, negative-sense single-stranded RNA viruses.[2] HeV is considered a high-consequence, highly pathogenic virus characterized by high mortality rates in humans (57%) and horses (80%).[3,4] HeV first emerged in Australia in 1994 and is classified as a biosafety level (BSL)-4 organism, which is the highest level of biocontainment.[3] HeV infection is a notifiable disease in all states and territories of Australia.[5] Severe respiratory and neurological symptoms occur in horses from HeV. HeV is an important zoonotic

School of Veterinary Science, The University of Queensland, Gatton Campus, Building 8114, Inner Ring Road, Gatton, Queensland 4343, Australia
* Corresponding author.
E-mail address: allison.stewart@uq.edu.au

Vet Clin Equine 39 (2023) 89–98
https://doi.org/10.1016/j.cveq.2022.11.009
0749-0739/23/© 2022 Elsevier Inc. All rights reserved.

disease in Australia, as humans have been infected secondarily from horses leading to severe illness and even death.

Natural hosts of HeV in Australia include the black flying fox (*Pteropus alecto*), the grey headed flying fox (*Pteropus poliocephalus*), the spectacled flying fox (*Pteropus conspicillatus*), and the little red flying fox (*Pteropus scapulatus*).[6,7] Epidemiologically, *P alecto* is considered the most important species, followed by *P conspicillatus*, because shedding of the main HeV variant has been demonstrated from these species.[4,8] Horses act as an amplifying host and are the only known mammalian species that has been infected directly from bats. Direct (ocular/nasal or oral mucous membrane contact when horses are resting or browsing under trees in which flying-foxes roost) or indirect contact (pasture or feed contaminated) with flying-fox urine is thought to be the main route of transmission of the disease from bats to horses.[8–10] Other body fluids, such as aborted fetuses, or associated fetal fluid, blood, feces, nasal discharge, and saliva are less likely but potential transmission sources.[10–13] Infected horses can spread the virus through aerosol transmission to other horses and humans.[7] So far, humans have only been infected directly from horses and not from bats or other humans. Horse-to-horse and horse-to-human transmissions are likely through contact with infected bodily fluids, especially nasal or oral secretions, from an infected horse during all stages of disease from preclinical to postmortem.[14]

To date, 2 asymptomatic dogs have been naturally infected from exposure to infected horses.[15–17] Although HeV is not highly pathogenic for dogs, it is strongly suggested that dogs should be kept away from infected horses. The 2 asymptomatic dogs were subjected to euthanasia to minimize the risk of viral transmission.[14,18] The risk of transmission of HeV from infected dogs to other domestic species, including humans, remains unknown.[15] Experimental infection has been successful in dogs,[19] pigs,[20] hamsters,[21] guinea pigs,[22–24] ferrets,[25] African green monkeys,[26] cats,[24,27] and horses.[14] Notwithstanding the very high viral doses used in experimental inoculations, dogs, cats, guinea pigs, ferrets, and pigs housed outdoors are plausible susceptible hosts of HeV infection and may conceivably transmit the virus to humans.[3]

EPIDEMIOLOGY

HeV was first identified in 1994 at a racing stable in the Brisbane suburb of Hendra, with 14 horses dying of acute severe respiratory illness.[28] There were 2 human close contacts, the trainer and a stable hand, who became unwell. The trainer died after 6 days in intensive care, and the stable hand survived. Retrospectively, an additional human death (husband of a veterinarian who performed a field necropsy near Mackay in Queensland [QLD]) was diagnosed with relapsing encephalitis and died 13 months after exposure to respiratory secretions of 2 infected horses.[29] During the past 28 years, there have been 66 spillover events with 108 horses having died or been subjected to euthanasia and 7 humans infected. Four of the infected people died as a consequence of the disease, with some of the survivors experiencing permanent long-term sequelae.[30]

The majority of the outbreaks happened in the autumn or winter months (between June and September) in southeast QLD and northeast New South Wales (NSW) regions.[31] In 2011, there were 18 spillover events with 24 horses involved followed by 8 outbreaks in 2012. The last spillover occurred in Mackay, QLD in early July 2022, which involved a 21-year-old unvaccinated horse, which demonstrated only neurological signs (staggering) with muzzle edema. The horse was subjected to euthanasia after its condition rapidly deteriorated.[32]The natural mortality rate in horses remains undetermined because all horses that test positive have previously been subjected to euthanasia to prevent further spreading of the virus to either horses or humans. Among infected humans, the veterinary profession is overly represented (4 of 7 cases) and is considered a high-risk group for the disease.[7] In addition to the 3 infected veterinarians and 1 veterinary nurse, the husband of a veterinarian, who assisted with a necropsy on an HeV-infected horse became infected and later died. Extreme caution should be taken when performing invasive diagnostic, treatment or necropsy procedures of horses with suspected HeV infections.[3]

HeV variants include prototype HeV (HeV-g1) and a novel variant genotype 2 (HeV-g2), which was detected in the spillover event in NSW in October 2021. The new variant HeV-g2 was then identified in archived samples from a 12-year-old Arabian gelding from QLD who was severely ill in 2015 and was suspected of having HeV and subjected to euthanasia but initially tested negative to HeV-g1.[10] Although HeV-g1 has been detected in tissues of all 4 flying fox species, only *P Alecto* and *P conspicillatus* excrete the virus, suggesting these 2 species are the primary sources of transmission to horses.[7,8] In addition to the 2 spillover events in NSW and QLD, the new variant HeV-g2 has also been detected in *P alecto* and *P poliocephalus* flying foxes from samples collected from NSW and QLD,[8] as well as in *P poliocephalus* flying foxes from samples collected from Victoria and South Australia and one *P scapulatus* flying fox sample from Western Australia indicating the level of genetic diversity for HeV is broader than first recognized.[33] These studies also demonstrate that there is a risk of spillover events in a much broader geographical area than what was first described.[8,33] Pteropid bats are a highly mobile species, and these studies demonstrate widespread shedding of the HeV prototype (HeV-g1) and novel variant genotype (HeV-g2), and therefore, HeV infections in horses should be considered in any horse with consistent history and clinical signs in Australia.[34]

The survival of HeV within the environment is longer in winter than in summer. Virus survival is also greater at higher latitudes irrespective of the time of year.[35] Environmental survival of HeV is highly sensitive to temperature and desiccation. The half-life of the virus is usually limited to a few hours; however, under optimal conditions it can survive for a couple of days.[36]

CLINICAL FEATURES

Bats infected with HeV seem to be asymptomatic.[37] The incubation period of HeV in horses is between 4 and 16 days, and in experimentally infected horses, shedding of virus occurred up to 5 days before development of clinical signs.[38] There are no clinical signs pathognomonic for HeV infection in horses, and clinical signs are often nonspecific and variable. However, HeV infection is often characterized by rapid deterioration in acutely affected horses. Horses infected with HeV predominately demonstrate clinical signs related to the respiratory and neurological systems, although nonspecific early signs such as fever, depression, inappetence, and restlessness are very common (**Table 1**).[3,7,31] Fever and an increased heart rate were the earliest signs in experimentally infected horses.[22] Neurological manifestations of the disease include ataxia, disorientation, head tilt, facial nerve paralysis, circling, and seizures.[31,39] Labored breathing, tachypnea, frothy or blood-tinged nasal or oral discharges are not uncommon terminal signs with respiratory involvement. Sudden death and colic have also been reported.[7,31]

SUMMARY OF CLINICAL SIGNS FROM LABORATORY...

HeV causes similar pathologic condition in different species as the virus shares the same virus entry receptor, Ephrin-B2, which is expressed on neurons, smooth muscle,

Table 1
Clinical signs summarization from laboratory testing submission forms or media releases since 1994 (Not all information for all cases was accessible to Biosecurity QLD)[31]

Clinical Signs	Number of Cases (n)	Percentage (%)
Nonspecific clinical signs (depressed, lethargic, inapparent)	48	56
Neurological signs (ataxia, disorientation, wide-based stance)	42	49
Fever	24	28
Respiratory signs (increased respiratory rate or effort)	22	26
Blood-stained frothy nasal/oral discharge	21	25
Elevated heart rate	17	20
Sudden death	15	18
Muscle twitching	7	8
Blindness	5	6
Colic	4	5
Facial swelling	4	5

and endothelial cells surrounding small arteries. Pathologic condition of acute henipavirus infection in humans is characterized by disseminated small vessel vasculopathy and parenchymal lesions in multiple major organs, such as the central nervous system, lung, and kidney. The most frequent gross lesions in horses have been found in the lower respiratory tract including dilated pulmonary lymphatics, severe pulmonary edema, and congestion. In several horses, there was nonsuppurative encephalitis characterized by perivascular cuffing of lymphocytes, neuronal necrosis, and focal gliosis.[40]

DIAGNOSIS

According to the national Australian guidelines, an animal is considered to be infected with HeV if polymerase chain reaction (PCR) or virus isolation (VI) or immunohistochemistry are positive. If an animal without any clinical signs tests positive, it is still considered a HeV-infected animal.[34]

Sampling

Use of personal protective equipment (PPE) is strictly mandated when handling horses suspected to be infected with HeV, especially when collecting samples for disease confirmation. Use of PPE is highly recommended on any sick horse (considering that the earliest clinical signs are depression and inappetence) that has not been adequately vaccinated against HeV anywhere in mainland Australia where flying foxes reside. This includes states where HeV spillover events have yet to be described.[3] An ethylenediamine tetraacetic acid (EDTA) blood sample and a nasal swab are the minimum recommended specimens required for confirmation of infection. Other samples that may be useful include oral, rectal, and vaginal swabs. Swabs taken from the ground soaked in freshly voided urine may be acceptable. Because positive HeV cases have had negative results from some submitted fluids, testing of multiple fluids is recommended to increase the chance of diagnosis. Similar samples can be collected from dead horses, with submission of blood clots and a dissected submandibular lymph node (chilled) acceptable without conducting a complete necropsy.[41] Performing necropsies on infected horses markedly increases the risk of transmission of the virus to humans (and other horses in the vicinity) and should not be performed on any horse where the death is potentially considered to be the result of HeV.[12] BSL-4 conditions are required when handling live HeV.[13] Diagnostic tests including PCR and enzyme-linked immunosorbent assay (ELISA) can be performed in a BSL-3 laboratory, whereas the virus neutralization test (VNT) and VI are only performed in BSL-4 laboratories.[41,42]

Methods of Virus Detection

Due to the fulminant and lethal course of the disease, PCR and VI are used for definitive diagnosis of acute infection. PCR is the primary recommended test for the acutely sick horses and can be conducted on a range of different types of samples (blood, blood clots, swabs, and tissue samples) with a result obtained within 4 hours. An updated quantitative reverse transcription-PCR has recently been applied to routine priority detection of the novel HeV variant (HeV-g2) in many animal and human health laboratories in Australia.[8,10,31]

Serology

Both ELISA and VNT tests detect the presence of HeV antibodies in serum samples and are typically used for titer testing of vaccinated horses.[16] A negative ELISA result indicates no exposure to HeV previously while a positive ELISA result requires differentiation of infected and vaccinated animals (DIVAs) to definitively differentiate past infections from the production of neutralizing anti-G antibodies from vaccination. Virus neutralization test and DIVA testing can only be performed at the Australian Centre for Disease Preparedness (ACDP; Newcomb, Victoria, Australia). A new indirect enzyme-linked assay (iELISA) using a recombinantly expressed HeV soluble G glycoprotein (HeV-sG iELASA) has been developed to replace the previously used HeV iELISA. The sensitivity (Se) of the new test is 84.2% with a higher specificity (Sp) of 97.1% compared with the previous HeV iELISA. Almost all false-positive results can be eliminated using the new test.[17] According to the World Organization for Animal Health (formerly, Office International des Épizooties) recommendations, a positive or nonspecific sera from ELISA from a suspect case should be followed by confirmatory test (VNT).[17] Ideally, serology should not be used as a lone diagnostic tool in cases of suspect HeV as PCR is the gold standard for virus detection. Because ELISA tests use inactivated virus, they can be performed in PC2 or PC3 laboratories; however, the VNT uses live virus and must be performed in a BSL-4 laboratory.[3]

A microsphere immune-assay (Luminex assay) has also been designed to detect antibodies against henipaviruses.[2] The assays are designed in total antibody binding (designed for antibody detection and differentiation) and restricted receptor-blocking formats (designed as a surrogate for virus neutralization; binding assay Se = 95.24%, Sp = 99.64%; blocking assay Se = 95.24%, Sp = 100%).[16] In the binding assay, bound antibody is detected using biotinylated Protein A together with biotinylated Protein G. For the receptor-blocking assay, the presence of HeV antibodies in the serum is detected by the ability to block biotinylated Ephrin B2. Both assays are read using a Bio-Plex Protein Assay System integrated with Bio-Plex Manager Software (Bio-Rad Laboratories, Hercules, CA, USA) for data acquisition and analysis.[16] Luminex assays have been shown to be rapid, sensitive in detecting HeV antibody in horses, and the tests do not require BSL-4 containment.

MANAGEMENT OF HeV-INFECTED ANIMALS

The Australian Veterinary Emergency Plan created by Animal Health Australia is a national response strategy for HeV.[34] It dictates that a risk assessment should be performed on a case-by-case basis by the state or territory Chief Veterinary Officer (CVO) to determine an appropriate management plan for all confirmed cases of HeV in horses. This risk assessment considers the animal welfare, human health risk, and the wishes of the owner. The risk assessment is also made in consultation with the jurisdictional human health department. In the majority of cases, the infected horses are subjected to euthanasia because of animal welfare concerns. The jurisdictional CVO may also decide to subject an infected animal to euthanasia to limit further transmission of HeV. In cases where the transmission risks, as well as the animal welfare, can be safely managed, the CVO may decide that veterinary supportive care and treatment is feasible. In situations where veterinary management of a HeV-positive animal is considered, the following requirements must be adhered to:

- The HeV-infected animal must be separated from nonclinical animals to limit horizontal transmission. For horses, a fenced yard or stable with a minimum 5-meter buffer from susceptible species is required.
- Quarantine and movement controls are imposed on the property for a minimum of 20 days.
- Personnel should use strategies that minimize the need for frequent contact.
- Animals that survive require serological testing 20 days following the onset of clinical signs to detect the presence of antibody. PCR testing should also be repeated until a negative result is returned. Then once the CVO has determined that the animal has clinically recovered and at least 20 days have elapsed since the onset of clinical signs, the quarantine can be removed.[34]

To date, all horses that have been positively identified as infected with HeV have been subjected to euthanasia due to animal welfare concerns, biosecurity concerns, and the potential for horizontal transmission.

Humans affected by HeV infection demonstrate acute respiratory illness and/or relapsing encephalitis.[19,43] In one HeV patient, relapsing encephalitis ultimately led to death 13 months after an initial diagnosis of aseptic meningitis. Self-limiting influenza-like illness (fever, myalgia, and headache) occurred in 3 of the infected survivors.[20] In some cases, influenza-like illness progressed to encephalitis.[7]

There is no licensed anti-HeV therapeutic for use in any species.[21] Ribavirin administered at an initial dose of 30 mg/kg followed by 15 g/kg every 6 hours intravenously has been used on infected humans although the activity of ribavirin against HeV is uncertain.[23] Monoclonal antibodies (mAbs) are under development and have been used as postexposure prophylaxis (PEP) against HeV in 16 human cases.[10] The furthest in development is mAb m102.4, which has phase 1 data showing safety, tolerability, intended pharmacokinetics, and no immunogenicity.[24,25] Combinations of cross-reactive humanized fusion (F) protein and receptor-binding protein mAbs have also been described for clinical development as PEP.[10,25]

PREVENTION OF HeV

Management changes can be implemented to limit the exposure of horses to flying foxes in an attempt to prevent HeV spillover events. These may include housing horses exclusively indoors, or at least placing feed bins and water troughs under cover and away from areas where flying foxes feed or roost. At a minimum, flowering and fruiting tress on the property, which attract flying foxes, should be identified and horses should be removed from these paddocks. However, it should be remembered that vaccination of horses is the single most effective preventative measure against HeV.[26,34]

Vaccination

The first (and only) HeV equine vaccine, Equivac HeV, was launched in November 2012 under permit and then registered in 2015 by Pfizer Animal Health (now Zoetis).

The strategy of equine vaccination was to prevent transmission of the virus in horses, and thus, indirectly protect humans.[27] It is a subunit vaccine, which contains recombinant HeV soluble G (sG) glycoprotein. This was the first vaccine commercialized against a BSL-4 agent and currently is the only commercially licensed prophylactic treatment of HeV. There is no commercially available vaccine for humans; however, a human vaccine based on the same immunogen as Equivac HeV using HeV-sG is now in phase 1 clinical trials.[25]

The vaccine contains not less than 100 μg of HeV-sG glycoprotein antigen adjuvanted with 250 μg/dose of immune-stimulating complex and a preservative in a 1 mL dose. The vaccine is administered by intramuscular injection.[44] It is recommended that horses aged older than 4 months commence the vaccination schedule, with the first 2 doses given 3 to 6 weeks apart and a third dose 6 months after the second, followed by annual boosters. Pregnant mares should not be vaccinated during the first 45 days of gestation or 2 weeks before parturition. Vaccination of foals born to vaccinated mares should have their primary series of vaccines delayed and commence the vaccination schedule at 6 months of age. It is recommended that a microchip be implanted and the animal identified before administration of the first vaccination. The microchip ID, vaccine batch number, date of administration, and recipient details are entered into an online registry at https://www.zoetis.com.au/vets-australia. The Hendra vaccination registry is used to help veterinarians, owners, and event organizers determine the HeV vaccination status of individual horses. Only veterinarians are permitted to register HeV vaccination of individual horses, and it is imperative that the information entered into the system is accurate.[12] Concerningly, a low percentage (11%–17%) of horses in Australia is HeV vaccinated.[45] Vaccination cost, safety, and effectiveness have been raised as concerns for horse owners. Therefore, trust and communication between veterinarians and their clients is important to educate owners of the risk of HeV infection.[45] Titer tests have been requested by many horse owners as an alternative to annual vaccination. The VNT can be used to detect antibodies after vaccination. The test can only be conducted at ACDP and is more expensive (US$367 per test in 2020[46]) than the vaccination. In an experimental study, horses that had an HeV titer of 1:16 or greater did not develop clinical signs and survived while unvaccinated horses succumbed to infection.[21,39] A titer cutoff of 64 is considered as protective by the majority of veterinarians even if vaccination has lapsed.[46]

Biosecurity

HeV poses a severe concern to public health, and infected horses can initially show mild and nonspecific clinical signs. It is critical for individual veterinarians and veterinary clinics to implement protocols to minimize the possibility of disease transmission and identify infected patients as soon as possible. Some veterinary hospitals in Australia have adopted protocols such that they will not admit horses without a valid HeV vaccination certificate or negative HeV exclusion result. Examples of HeV hospital protocols (strict and less rigorous) have been previously described in detail.[3]

HeV vaccination status of an individual horse can be determined online via the Hendra vaccination registry (https://www.health4horses.com.au/). The implanted microchip should be scanned and must match the information on the HeV vaccination certificate. Precautions must still be taken with any horse showing clinical signs that may be related to HeV infection, even in the face of valid proof of vaccination as no vaccine is 100% effective in all recipients. PPE including face shield, P2 mask, disposable gown, gloves, and shoe covers must be worn when dealing with suspicious horses.[3] In a strict biosecurity protocol, horses without a valid HeV vaccination record should undergo a HeV exclusion test using EDTA blood before admittance to the clinic.[3]

Veterinarians who fail to restrict access or treat any horses that subsequently test positive to HeV may face a workplace health and safety fine of US$10,000, with potential for revocation of their veterinary license and civil liability lawsuits.[3] If HeV is a differential, no further diagnostic or laboratory testing or intensive medical or surgical treatment can be performed except for taking samples for HeV exclusion testing and administering analgesics while wearing full PPE.

FUTURE RESEARCH

Due to the highly infectious and deadly nature of the virus and the mandate implemented before 2016 that any horse infected with HeV is subjected to euthanasia, endeavors to conduct studies focusing on treatment or survival are prevented.[34] As a BSL-4 organism, only a limited number of laboratories can perform research on the organism after strict approval processes.

So far 2 HeV variants HeV-g1 and HeV-g2 have been detected, with the likelihood of further variants being present or evolving. Climate change and flying fox habitat destruction may result in further spillover events in more diverse locations. Therefore, virus-detection testing must continue to evolve and vigilance encouraged throughout mainland Australia.

The Equivac HeV vaccine is considered as safe and effective to protect horses, and therefore, humans. To date, all recorded HeV cases have involved adult horses with the exception of one foal of 5 months of age.[31] No studies have been conducted on foals. It is assumed that foals born from vaccinated mares would be protected from maternal antibodies but the variability and duration of protection requires further investigation.

REFERENCES

1. Calisher CH, Childs JE, Field HE, et al. Bats: important reservoir hosts of emerging viruses. Clin Microbiol Rev 2006;19(3):531–45.
2. Bossart KN, McEachern JA, Hickey AC, et al. Neutralization assays for differential henipavirus serology using Bio-Plex protein array systems. J Virol Methods 2007; 142(1–2):29–40.
3. Yuen KY, Fraser NS, Henning J, et al. Hendra virus: Epidemiology dynamics in relation to climate change, diagnostic tests and control measures. One Health 2021;12:100207.
4. Goldspink LK, Edson DW, Vidgen ME, et al. Natural Hendra Virus Infection in Flying-Foxes - Tissue Tropism and Risk Factors. PLoS One 2015;10(6):e0128835.
5. Halpin K, Young PL, Field HE, et al. Isolation of Hendra virus from pteropid bats: a natural reservoir of Hendra virus. J Gen Virol 2000;81(8):1927–32.
6. Iehlé C, Razafitrimo G, Razainirina J, et al. Henipavirus and tioman virus antibodies in pteropodid bats, Madagascar. Emerg Infect Dis 2007;13(1):159–61.
7. Halpin K Rota P. A review of Hendra Virus and Nipah Virus Infections in Man and other Animals. Zoonoses-Infections Affecting Humans Anim Springer Netherlands, 2014;997–1012.
8. Peel AJ, Yinda CK, Annand EJ, et al. Novel Hendra virus Variant Circulating in Black Flying Foxes and Grey-Headed Flying Foxes. Australia, Emerging Infect Dieseases 2022;28:1043–7.
9. Field HE. Hendra virus ecology and transmission. Curr Opin Virol 2016;16:120–5.

10. Annand EJ, Horsburgh BA, Xu K, et al. Novel hendra virus variant detected by sentinel surveillance of horses in Australia. Emerg Infect Dis 2022;28(3):693–704.

11. Edson D, Field H, McMichael L, et al. Routes of hendra virus excretion in naturally-infected flying-foxes: implications for viral transmission and spillover risk. PLoS One 2015;10(10):e0140670.

12. Halpin K, Graham K, Durr PA, et al. Sero-monitoring of horses demonstrates the equivac((R)) hev hendra virus vaccine to be highly effective in inducing neutralising antibody titres. Vaccines (Basel) 2021;9(7):731.

13. Fischer K, Diederich S, Smith G, et al. Indirect ELISA based on Hendra and Nipah virus proteins for the detection of henipavirus specific antibodies in pigs. PLoS One 2018;13(4):e0194385.

14. Middleton DJ, Riddell S, Klein R, et al. Experimental Hendra virus infection of dogs: virus replication, shedding and potential for transmission. Aust Vet J 2017;95(1–2):10–8.

15. Kirkland PD, Gabor M, Poe I, et al. Hendra virus infection in dog, Australia, 2013. Emerg Infect Dis 2015;21(12):2182–5.

16. McNabb L, Barr J, Crameri G, et al. Henipavirus microsphere immuno-assays for detection of antibodies against Hendra virus. J Virol Methods 2014;200:22–8.

17. Colling A, Lunt R, Bergfeld J, et al. A network approach for provisional assay recognition of a Hendra virus antibody ELISA: test validation with low sample numbers from infected horses. J Vet Diagn Invest 2018;30(3):362–9.

18. Australian veterinary emergency plan 2013, https://www.qldhorsecouncil.com/QldHorseCouncil/media/QHC-Portal/Hendra%20Virus/Hendra-EAD-Response-Policy-Brief.pdf.

19. O'Sullivan JD, Sullivan JD, Allowrth AM, Paterson DL, et al. Fatal encephalitis due to novel paramyxovirus transmitted from horses. Lancet 1997;349(9045):93–5.

20. Hanna JN, McBride WJ, Brookes DL, et al. Hendra virus infection in a veterinarian. Med J Aust 2006;185(10):562–4.

21. Middleton D, Pallister J, Klein R, et al. Hendra virus vaccine, a one health approach to protecting horse, human, and environmental health. Emerg Infect Dis 2014;20(3):372–9.

22. Hendra virus infection, Available at: https://www.cfsph.iastate.edu/Factsheets/pdfs/hendra.pdf, 2015.

23. Playford EG, McCall B, Smith G, et al. Human Hendra virus encephalitis associated with equine outbreak, Australia, 2008. Emerg Infect Dis 2010;16(2):219–23.

24. Gómez Román R, Tornieporth N, Cherian NG, et al. Medical countermeasures against henipaviruses: a review and public health perspective. Lancet Infect Dis 2022;22(1):e13–27.

25. Geisbert TW, Bobb K, Borisevich V, et al. A single dose investigational subunit vaccine for human use against Nipah virus and Hendra virus. NPJ Vaccin 2021;6(1):23.

26. Hendra virus – information for horse businesses, Available at: https://www.worksafe.qld.gov.au/__data/assets/pdf_file/0028/16597/hendra-virus-horse.pdf, 2018.

27. Broder CC, Xu K, Nikolov DB, et al. A treatment for and vaccine against the deadly Hendra and Nipah viruses. Antivir Res 2013;100(1):8–13.

28. Murray K, Selleck P, Hopper P, et al. A morbillivirus that caused fatal disease in horses and humans. Science 1995;268(5207):94–7.

29. Summary of human cases of Hendra virus infection, Available at https://www.health.nsw.gov.au/Infectious/controlguideline/Pages/hendra-case-summary.aspx, 2022.

30. Taylor C, Playford EG, McBride WJH, et al. No evidence of prolonged Hendra virus shedding by 2 patients, Australia. Emerg Infect Dis 2012;18(12):2025–7.

31. Summary of Hendra virus incidents in horses, Available at: https://www.business.qld.gov.au/industries/service-industries-professionals/service-industries/veterinary-surgeons/guidelines-hendra/incident-summar, 2022. Accessed July 22, 2022.

32. Hendra virus detected in Mackay horse, Abailable at. https://www.daf.qld.gov.au/news-media/media-centre/biosecurity/news/hendra-virus-detected-in-mackay-horse.

33. Wang J, Anderson DE, Halpin K, et al. A new Hendra virus genotype found in Australian flying foxes. Virol J 2021;18(1):197.

34. Australian veterinary emergency plan, Available at https://animalhealthaustralia.com.au/wp-content/uploads/dlm_uploads/2021/07/AVP_RS_HendraVirus_V5.pdf, 2021.

35. Scanlan JC, Kung NY, Selleck PW, et al. Survival of hendra virus in the environment: modelling the effect of temperature. Ecohealth 2015;12(1):121–30.

36. Fogarty R, Halpin K, Hyatt AD, et al. Henipavirus susceptibility to environmental variables. Virus Res 2008;132(1–2):140–4.

37. Halpin K, Hyatt AD, Fogarty R, et al. Pteropid bats are confirmed as the reservoir hosts of henipaviruses: A comprehensive experimental study of virus transmission. Am J Trop Med Hyg 2011;85(5):946–51.

38. Baldock F, Douglas I, Halpin K, et al. Epidemiological investigations into the 1994 equine morbillivirus outbreaks in Queensland, Australia. Singapore Vet J 1996;20:57–61.

39. Field H, Schaaf K, Kung N, et al. Hendra virus outbreak with novel clinical features, Australia. Emerg Infect Dis 2010;16(2):338–40.

40. Lee B Rota P A, Rota PA. Henipavirus. 1. Aufl. ed., 359. Berlin, Heidelberg: Springer-Verlag; 2012.

41. Hendra virus sampling, submission and testing, Available at https://www.business.qld.gov.au/industries/service-industries-professionals/service-industries/veterinary-surgeons/guidelines-hendra/sampling-tests, 2018.

42. Feldman KS, Foord A, Heine HG, et al. Design and evaluation of consensus PCR assays for henipaviruses. J Virol Methods 2009;161(1):52–7.

43. Selvey LA, Wells RM, McCormack JG, et al. Infection of humans and horses by a newly described morbillivirus. Med J Aust 1995;162(12):642–5.

44. Tan R, Hodge A, Klein R, et al. Virus-neutralising antibody responses in horses following vaccination with Equivac(R) HeV: a field study. Aust Vet J 2018;96(5):161–6.

45. Manyweathers J, Field H, Longnecker N, et al. "Why won't they just vaccinate" Horse owner risk perception and uptake of the Hendra virus vaccine. BMC Vet Res 2017;13(1):103.

46. Barrett RS, Wiethoelter A, Halpin K. The Hendra virus vaccine: perceptions regarding the role of antibody titre testing. Aust Vet J 2021;99(9):412–8.

Eastern, Western, and Venezuelan Equine Encephalitis and West Nile Viruses
Clinical and Public Health Considerations

Daniela Luethy, DVM, MPH, DACVIM*

KEYWORDS

- Flavivirus • Alphavirus • Arbovirus • Horse • Mosquito-borne disease • Encephalitis
- Neurologic

KEY POINTS

- Mosquito-borne viral diseases are the most common infection of the equine central nervous system globally and are increasingly more common as the spatiotemporal distribution of the vector increases.
- The clinical signs of the various encephalitis viruses can overlap significantly, which can present a challenge for the clinician.
- Veterinary practitioners should be aware of the continued emergence of alphavirus and flavivirus infections and the interconnectedness between human and equine health.

INTRODUCTION

From the identification of Western Equine Encephalitis Virus (WEEV) in the brain of an encephalitic horse in California in 1930, to the global spread of West Nile Virus (WNV) in the late 1990s, our understanding of the epizootiology of mosquito-borne equine encephalitic viruses has grown, corresponding to an increasing incidence of disease. The emergence and spread of these diseases have also highlighted a growing public health concern.[1–3] With the progression of climate change, mosquito-borne disease transmission has and will continue to increase, driven by a greater spatiotemporal distribution of the vector.[2–6] A thorough understanding of these diseases is essential for the equine veterinary practitioner, but also for physicians and public health officials. This article describes equine encephalitis viruses with a focus on clinical and public health considerations. The reader is directed to the previous Veterinary Clinics article on these viruses for additional background information on pathophysiology.[7]

Large Animal Internal Medicine, Large Animal Clinical Sciences, College of Veterinary Medicine, University of Florida, PO Box 100136, Gainesville, FL 32610, USA
* Corresponding author.
E-mail address: dluethy@ufl.edu

Vet Clin Equine 39 (2023) 99–113
https://doi.org/10.1016/j.cveq.2022.11.007
0749-0739/23/Published by Elsevier Inc.

vetequine.theclinics.com

Abbreviations	
CSF	Cerebrospinal fluid
ELISA	Enzyme-linked immunosorbent assay
NSAID	Non-steroidal anti-inflammatory drug
DMSO	Dimethyl sulfoxide
IgM	Immunoglobulin M
EPM	Equine protozoal myeloencephalitis
EHM	Equine herpesvirus myeloencephalopathy
WNV	West Nile virus
WNE	West Nile encephalomyelitis
EEE	Eastern equine encephalitis
WEE	Western equine encephalitis
VEE	Venezuelan equine encephalitis

Although Western, Eastern, Venezuelan Equine Encephalitis Virus (VEEV), and WNV are the most commonly isolated viruses from encephalitic horses, many additional encephalitis viruses have been reported and their geographic distribution may increase in the future. In the *Alphavirus* family, in addition to Eastern equine encephalitis virus (EEEV), WEEV, and VEEV, Ross River virus in Australia and Papua New Guinea and Semliki Forest Virus in Africa have both been reported to cause neurologic disease in horses. In the *Flavivirus* family, additional equine viruses of note in North America include St. Louis encephalitis virus and Powassan virus. In addition, several viruses in the *Bunyavirus* family, including California encephalitis, Jamestown Canyon, La Crosse, and Snowshoe hare viruses, have been reported to cause encephalomyelitis in horses in North America.[7]

WEST NILE VIRUS
Etiology and Epidemiology

WNV is a positive-sense, single-stranded RNA *flavivirus* transmitted by mosquitoes.[8,9] WNV is a member of the Japanese B Encephalitis family of neuroinvasive arboviruses within the *Flavivirus* genus.[10] This family also includes Japanese encephalitis virus, Kunjin virus, and Murray Valley encephalitis virus, which have caused encephalomyelitis in horses outside North America.[10,11] There are seven genetic lineages of WNV and two of these have been associated with neuroinvasive disease in humans and horses. Lineage 1 is associated with outbreaks of human and equine neuroinvasive infections in the Mediterranean basin, West Africa, northern Europe, and North America. Lineage 2 is widespread in sub-Saharan Africa and was originally associated with subclinical equine infections, but since 2005, neuroinvasive infections associated with lineage 2 have been increasing in Africa and Europe.[12,13]

WNV is sustained in an enzootic cycle between mosquitoes and vertebrates, mainly birds.[9] Mosquitoes are the natural vectors of WNV, with over 150 species of mosquitoes capable of carrying WNV. *Culex spp.* are the major vectors, but the specific mosquito species varies by region, with *Culex pipiens* in the northeastern United States and *Culex tarsalis* in the western United States accounting for more than half of mosquito-positive pools.[14–17] Over 300 bird species have been identified as reservoir hosts of WNV, with the Corvidae family (which includes crows, ravens, and magpies) being the most important host, owing to their highly efficient viral amplification, and therefore, high levels of viremia.[18] Horses and humans achieve inadequate viremia to maintain the virus cycle and are incapable of virus amplification, making them "dead-end" accidental hosts.[9] Sheep and New World camelids can also develop neurologic disease after WNV exposure, and alligators may represent an important reservoir in the southeastern United States.[19–22] West Nile encephalitis cases mirror mosquito vector activity, which can be seasonal in temperate regions or year-round in tropical and subtropical areas.[3,23,24]

Clinical and Pathologic Findings

Most equine WNV infections are asymptomatic. Approximately 20% of infected horses will develop clinical signs and <10% develop myeloencephalitis.[25] Clinical outbreaks suggest a 1- to 2-week incubation period from infection to onset of clinical signs.[26] Mild to moderate fever is common, although it is possible that the fever has occurred before the veterinary examination, and therefore, is missed in a subset of horses. In WNV encephalomyelitis (WNE), motor deficits are asymmetric and multifocal, with signs attributable to polioencephalomyelitis, including primarily limb ataxia and weakness, with muzzle twitching, obtundation, recumbency, hyperesthesia/ hyperresponsiveness, and muscle fasciculations.[27–32] In addition, less common signs include dog-sitting posture, thoracic limb collapse, compulsive walking, muscle atrophy, seizure, circling, blindness, or head pressing.[26–32] Clinical signs often correlate with the predominance of lesions in the gray matter of the hindbrain and spinal cord, with the rostral brainstem and forebrain less commonly affected.[29] Owing to a predilection for gray matter in the thoracic spinal cord, some horses will present with acute-onset bilateral thoracic limb weakness or collapse with normal pelvic limb strength (**Fig. 1**A).[26] Horses may also have difficulty standing due to profound weakness (**Fig. 1**B). Neurologic clinical signs can vary from fairly mild, with only fine muzzle twitching, to rapid recumbency and death more reminiscent of EEE. Coarse muzzle twitching is a particular finding seen in many acute cases of WNE in horses, and muscle fasciculations and hyperesthesia are also very common.[26]

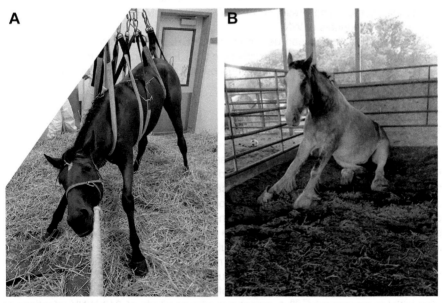

Fig. 1. (*A*) 2-year-old Standardbred filly diagnosed with West Nile Virus encephalomyelitis. This horse showed bilateral thoracic limb weakness and obtundation (Courtesy of Daniela Luethy, DVM). (*B*). 3-year-old Shire filly diagnosed with WNV encephalomyelitis, demonstrating dog-sitting posture due to weakness. (1*B* - Courtesy of Kallie Hobbs, DVM)

Complete blood count and serum biochemistry changes are often mild and nonspecific. Many affected horses will have pleocytosis on cerebrospinal fluid (CSF) cytologic analysis, often mononuclear, and mild xanthochromia is common. In a population of 30 horses in Florida, CSF nucleated cell counts ranged from 0 to 882/μL and CSF protein ranged from 64 to 316 mg/dL, and in a study of 35 horses, 77% had abnormal CSF with either mononuclear pleocytosis, high protein, or both.[26,27]

Gross necropsy findings are often limited to congestion of the meninges and hemorrhagic foci in the brain and spinal cord. Histology may reveal multifocal lymphocytic polioencephalomyelitis of variable severity, with a predominance in the ventral and lateral horns of the thoracolumbar spinal cord. In the brain, there is lymphocytic perivascular cuffing and microgliosis of the medulla oblongata and pons, as well as in the basal nuclei, thalamus, and mesencephalon to a lesser extent. There may be evidence of neuronal degeneration in severe cases.[26,29]

Diagnosis

A presumptive diagnosis of WNE is often made based on clinical signs, particularly in regions where the virus is active, and if the horse is unvaccinated or incompletely vaccinated. The presence of muzzle twitching should increase the suspicion of WNE.[26] However, no pathognomonic signs exist and other differential diagnoses should be considered. A mild to moderate CSF mononuclear pleocytosis supports the diagnosis, although lack of this finding does not rule out the diagnosis (**Table 1**). In a horse with clinical signs of WNE, a positive serum IgM antibody-capture enzyme-linked immunosorbent assay (ELISA) and negative results of other tests (alphaviruses, herpesvirus, EPM, hepatic encephalopathy) supports a diagnosis of WNV infection; however, serum antibody tests only support diagnosis of WNV infection, not necessarily WNE.[33,34] Clinicians should remember that for each case of WNE, there are approximately nine horses with WNV infection with non-neurologic or subclinical infections.[26] The presence of WNV-specific IgM in CSF increases the test specificity for diagnosis of WNE.

Post-mortem diagnosis can be made using PCR, immunohistochemistry, or virus isolation to show viral components within the CNS. However, due to low viral load during WNV infection, detection of the virus by any modality, including PCR, can be unreliable.[35]

Treatment and Prognosis

There is no specific antiviral treatment for WNE and the mainstay of treatment is supportive care and anti-inflammatories. Supportive care should include secure footing, deep clean bedding, protection of bony prominences for recumbent horses, and adequate food and water. Sling support can be considered in some horses. Non-steroidal anti-inflammatory drugs (NSAIDs) are typically used for analgesia, anti-inflammatory effects, and anti-pyretic effects. Administration of corticosteroids is controversial. Dimethyl sulfoxide (DMSO), vitamin E, and pentoxifylline can be considered. Some WNE model studies as well as anecdotal evidence have suggested benefits of Type I interferons or interferon inducers and hyperimmune globulin products.

Recovery can take several months and not all horses will fully recover.[30] Between 10% and 40% of horses will have residual neurologic deficits.[30,36] Mortality from WNE is ~30% and approximately a third of horses may experience a relapse of signs after initial improvement.[27,36] A recent surveillance study of 842 WNV infections in horses in Canada from 2003 to 2019 found that 96% of cases occurred in unvaccinated horses and the mortality risk was 31.9%.[37] Risk factors for mortality in horses include lack of vaccination, housing in pastures or with solid stall walls, light coat color,

Table 1
Common findings of Eastern Equine Encephalitis, Western Equine Encephalitis, Venezuelan Equine Encephalitis, and West Nile Viruses

	Eastern Equine Encephalitis Virus	Western Equine Encephalitis Virus	Venezuelan Equine Encephalitis Virus	West Nile Virus
Virus type	ssRNA	ssRNA	ssRNA	ssRNA
Major vector	Culiseta melanura, Aedes taeniorhynchus	Culex tarsalis, Culiseta melanura	Enzootic—Culex melanoconion spp. Epizootic—wide vector range	Many Culex spp.
Reservoir host	Passerine birds (rodents)	Passerine birds	Small rodents	Birds
Amplifying host	Passerine birds (rodents)	Passerine birds	Small rodents, horses	Birds
Clinical signs	Fever, obtundation, dementia, blindness, cranial nerve deficits, ataxia, paresis, recumbency, seizures EEE typically more severe and more rapid progression		Fever, ataxia, paresis, recumbency, seizures	Fever, ataxia, paresis, muscle fasciculations, muscle twitching
CSF color	Normal to mildly turbid	Normal	Similar to EEE/WEE	Mild xanthochromia
CSF protein	Elevated	Normal to mildly elevated	Similar to EEE/WEE	Normal to elevated
CSF white blood cell count	Elevated	Mildly elevated	Similar to EEE/WEE	Normal to elevated
CSF cell differential	Neutrophilic (most common) Mononuclear	Mononuclear	Similar to EEE/WEE	Mononuclear
Ante-mortem diagnostic test(s)	IgM Capture ELISA	IgM Capture ELISA, PRNT[a]	IgM Capture ELISA, PRNT[a]	IgM Capture ELISA
Treatment	Supportive care, anti-inflammatories, anti-convulsants, mannitol or hypertonic saline for cerebral edema			Supportive care, anti-inflammatories
Case fatality rate	75% to 90%	20% to 30%	19% to 83%	22% to 44%
Pathologic findings	Acute to subacute, multifocal to diffuse meningoencephalomyelitis, predominantly gray matter			Polioencephalomyelitis, meningeal congestion

Abbreviation: PRNT, plaque-reduction neutralizing titer.
[a] Not readily commercially-available.

and the use of stable fans.[38,39] There is conflicting evidence of a sex predilection.[30,32,38,39] Recumbent horses, no or incomplete vaccination, paresis of pelvic limbs, and facial/tongue paralysis are associated with a poor outcome.[27,30,32] Mortality rises with increasing age after 5 years.[27,30,32]

Prevention

Prevention consists of mosquito control and vaccination. Currently available vaccines include an inactivated whole virus vaccine, recombinant canarypox vector vaccine, and inactivated flavivirus chimera vaccine. Available WNV vaccines only include lineage 1 virus; however, studies have shown cross-protection against natural infections from lineage 2 strains.[40–42] Boosters should be administered before the active vector season. Veterinarians should follow label and national agency guidelines, with consideration for more frequent vaccination in regions of high local disease, vector activity, and/or exposure risk. A recent review discussed core vaccine guidelines and the current commercially available vaccines in North America.[42]

Public Health Focus

WNV is transmitted to humans by the bite of infected mosquitos, primarily *Culex* species. Approximately 70% to 80% of human WNV infections are asymptomatic. Symptomatic individuals develop an acute febrile illness, including headache, arthralgia, GI signs, and transient rash.[43] Less than 1% of infected individuals develop neuroinvasive disease.[43] As dead-end hosts, horses infected with WNV do not pose a risk of zoonotic transmission to people, nor vice versa. However, a high incidence of WNV infection in horses suggests a high level of WNV circulating transmission in the region, and therefore, higher risk for humans in an endemic area. Human-to-human WNV transmission has also been shown to occur after contaminated blood transfusion or organ transplantation and via vertical transmission through placenta and breast milk.[44–49]

EASTERN, WESTERN, AND VENEZUELAN EQUINE ENCEPHALITIS VIRUSES
Etiology and Epidemiology

EEEV, WEEV, and VEEV are members of the genus *Alphavirus* associated with encephalitis in domestic equids.[50] These viruses are single-stranded, positive-sense RNA viruses first identified in the 1930s.[50–53]

EEE and WEE viruses are maintained in an enzootic cycle between New World passerine birds and ornithophilic mosquitoes. There is also some evidence suggesting that rodents may be significant hosts of EEEV in South America and possibly Florida, and small ground mammals, such as squirrels, may be important reservoirs of WEEV.[54,55] *C. tarsalis* mosquitoes are the vectors responsible for maintenance and amplification of WEEV, whereas *Culiseta melanura* is the major vector responsible for EEEV.[56–59] *C. tarsalis* can transfer WEE from birds to humans and/or horses, whereas several bridging vectors, primarily *Aedes, Coquillettidia,* and *Culex*, are responsible for transfer of EEE from birds to horse or human.[52,60–62] EEEV is also capable of causing disease in cats, dogs, alpacas, llamas, swine, deer, and cattle, with deer becoming a potentially important species for EEEV surveillance.[63–69]

Encephalitis associated with EEEV or WEEV usually occurs in susceptible horses 2 to 3 weeks after entry into the bird population in a region, with human infections occurring a few weeks later. Epizootics usually occur in the summer and early fall, although cases can occur year-round in southeastern states.[70] Although there are differences in the ecology of EEEV between the southeastern and northeastern United States, high level of rainfall, standing surface water, bush cover, proximity and size of tree plantations, and immune status of hosts have all been identified as risk factors for equine and human infections.[70–75]

VEEV has several important differences from EEEV and WEEV. Birds do not play a significant role in amplification and maintenance of VEE; rather, VEE is maintained in an enzootic cycle between sylvatic rodents and mosquitoes.[76,77] The Everglades virus, a VEE subtype II virus found in Florida, cycles between *Culex* subspecies mosquitoes and wild rodents.[50,78] When the VEE virus mutates to a more pathogenic strain and infects equids, the epizootic cycle involving equids as amplifying and reservoir hosts begins.[78] Infected animals develop a high level of viremia, and equids are amplification hosts of the virus, a defining feature of epizootic VEEV. Rabbits, goats, sheep, and dogs can also become infected, with a high mortality rate.[50] VEEV remains an important human pathogen, with epidemics revealing the interconnectivity between human and equine health.

Over the past few decades, reports of WEE infection in both horses and humans have been limited, likely due to protective immunity in the equine population related to vaccination and subclinical exposures, and the enzootic activity of WEEV in the United States continues to appear to be declining.[7,79–81]

Clinical and Pathologic Findings

Young horses appear particularly susceptible to alphaviral encephalitis. Infected horses are generally not vaccinated for encephalitis viruses. Clinical signs of all three viral infections in horses are similar, but EEE infections typically result in more severe signs and more rapid progression than WEE or VEE. Three clinical syndromes are described in experimental models, with horses responding in any or all of the following ways: (1) subclinical infection with low-grade viremia and fever; (2) generalized febrile illness, with decreased appetite, tachycardia, depression, and/or diarrhea; and (3) clinical encephalomyelitis.[50,82–84]

Neurologic signs occur approximately 7 days to 2 weeks after infection and most deaths occur 2 to 3 days after onset of neurologic signs, with the course of disease varying between 2 and 14 days.[50,82–84] Neurologic signs can be variable but, in general, appear as diffuse or multifocal forebrain disease, with progression to brainstem and spinal cord involvement as the diseases progresses. Some horses may not be found until they are recumbent, comatose, or dead. The most common initial sign is obtundation. Horses can appear apathetic and can progress to further signs of dementia, including head pressing (**Fig. 2**), odontoprisis, irritability, hyperesthesia,

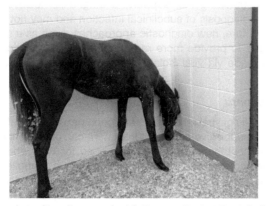

Fig. 2. Thoroughbred yearling diagnosed with Eastern Equine Encephalitis, demonstrating head pressing. (Courtesy of Martha Mallicote, DVM).

aggression, leaning, compulsive walking, and lack of menace response. Cranial nerve deficits can be seen as the disease progresses, and abnormal signs often start asymmetrically. Ataxia, paresis, and tremors may be seen. Physical examination abnormalities secondary to recumbency and trauma may also be seen.

Complete blood count and serum biochemistry changes are often mild and nonspecific. CSF cytologic analysis of horses with EEE is often abnormal, with high nucleated cell counts and high protein concentrations in many horses. In a referral population of horses in Florida, >95% of horses with EEE had abnormal CSF cytology, with 88% having high protein concentrations and 87% having high nucleated cell counts (range 0 to 3100/uL) with often a neutrophilic pleocytosis (Table 1).[50] Both nucleated cell counts and protein concentrations are typically higher in samples collected from the atlantooccipital space than lumbosacral; therefore, clinicians should consider their collection route when interpreting CSF results. In contrast to EEE, horses with WEE typically have a lymphocytic pleocytosis, with a range of nucleated cell counts from 12 to 30/uL.[50,85]

Gross necropsy findings often include congestion of most organs and a slate-gray discoloration of the brain and spinal cord with petechial hemorrhage. Histology reveals acute to subacute, multifocal to diffuse meningoencephalomyelitis, predominantly involving the gray matter, with diffuse neuronal degeneration, meningitis, perivascular as well as neuroparenchymal infiltrates, and gliosis.[50,82,85–87] Lesions are most severe in the cerebral cortex, thalamus, and hypothalamus.[85] Neutrophils predominate in acute EEE, with occasional eosinophils, whereas lymphocytes predominate in more chronic cases. Bronchopneumonia is seen in many fatal EEE cases, and myocardial necrosis may be seen, suggestive of brain-heart syndrome.[50]

Diagnosis

A presumptive diagnosis is often made based on clinical signs, particularly in regions where the virus is active and if the horse is unvaccinated or incompletely vaccinated. A CSF neutrophilic or lymphocytic pleocytosis supports a diagnosis of alphaviral encephalomyelitis. No reliable antemortem diagnostic test for detection of EEEV exists, and therefore, diagnosis relies on demonstration of immunoglobulin M (IgM). Serum IgM antibody capture-ELISA is the diagnostic test of choice.[72] If available, detection of CSF IgM antibody is more conclusive but horses often die before an intrathecal antibody response occurs.[85] If horses survive, a fourfold or higher increase between acute and convalescent titers via hemagglutination-inhibition or plaque-reduction neutralizing titer supports a diagnosis; however, positive results may only support a diagnosis of subclinical infection and may not confirm encephalomyelitis.[88] In the future, new diagnostic approaches, such as a multiplex serologic assay, may be used to provide more rapid pathogen identification.[89] Post-mortem diagnosis can be made via viral isolation, immunohistochemistry, or PCR of brain tissue.[90–93]

Treatment and Prognosis

No currently available antiviral medication has been proven to be effective. The mainstay of treatment is supportive care, and treatment can often be ineffective, particularly for EEE. Treatment is similar to that described for WNV above. Horses which are unable to stand should be euthanized. Seizures can be controlled with benzodiazepines or phenobarbital. Horses should be treated for cerebral edema and inflammation, with considerations for administration of NSAIDs, DMSO, and mannitol or hypertonic saline. Corticosteroids (dexamethasone) may be an important determinant of neurologic recovery in survivors.[50]

Case fatality rate is highest for EEE at 75% to 90%. Most horses can recover fully from WEE, with a case fatality rate of 20% to 30%, depending on the outbreak.[7,50] VEE is highly variable dependent on outbreak, with case fatality rate ranging from 19% to 83%.[50] Recovery can take months and some horses may retain residual neurologic deficits.

Prevention

Prevention consists of mosquito control and vaccination. EEE and WEE are 100% preventable using appropriate vaccination protocols.[7,42] Despite the dramatically declining incidence of WEE in the United States, WEE vaccination remains important because WEE infections continue to occur in Central and South America, and the potential for re-introduction into the United States exists, particularly if the equine population becomes immuno-naïve.[7,94] Only EEE and WEE vaccines are considered core vaccines in the United States.[42] VEE vaccines are not widely used in North America due to the potential for compromising international movement of horses.[85] Veterinarians should follow label and national agency guidelines, with consideration for more frequent vaccination in regions of high local disease, vector activity, and/or exposure risk. A recent review discussed core vaccine guidelines and the current commercially available vaccines in North America.[42] Although not currently recommended in North America, vaccination of horses for VEE in Central and South America should be considered, as a way to potentially eliminate VEEV epidemics, as horses can serve as the primary reservoir of the virus, and intensive research is ongoing in this area.[7,78,85] If widespread vaccination occurred in Central and South America, it is possible that VEE outbreaks could be prevented.[78]

Public Health Focus

Similar to WNV, alphaviruses are transmitted to humans by the bite of infected mosquitos. Although horses are dead-end hosts for EEEV and WEEV, they are amplifying hosts for VEEV and, therefore, play an important role in disease transmission.[43] Horses infected with EEEV or WEEV do not pose a risk of zoonotic transmission to people, nor vice versa, but a high incidence of EEEV or WEEV in horses may suggest a high level of these viruses in the region.[95] EEEV can be infectious to individuals handling CNS tissues or CSF, so precautions should be taken in horses where EEEV is suspected. In contrast to EEEV and WEEV, because horses are amplifying hosts for VEEV, some additional public health measures should be considered. These specific measures include determination of the extent of transmission by identifying infected horses and their human contacts, vaccination of all horses in and surrounding an affected region, and restriction of the movement of horses from affected areas.

The distribution of EEEV in North America has been expanding, with a concurrent increase in annual incidence of human infections.[60,61,95] Human mortality rates with EEEV approach 30%, with a large proportion of survivors suffering from chronic neurologic issues, resulting in significant personal and societal economic burden.[96] Because EEEV can also infect poultry, like turkey and quail, outbreaks can lead to significant economic and societal costs.[97]

SUMMARY

The continued recognition and emergence of alphavirus and flavivirus diseases is a growing veterinary and public health concern. As the global environment continues to change, mosquito-borne diseases will continue to evolve and expand. Continued development of readily available vaccines for prevention of these diseases in humans and animals is essential to controlling epizootics of these diseases. Further research into effective antiviral treatments is also sorely needed.

CLINICS CARE POINTS

- The clinical signs of the various encephalitis viruses can overlap significantly, which can present a challenge for the clinician. Although no clinical signs are pathognomonic for type of viral encephalitis, coarse muzzle twitching and hyperesthesia may increase suspicion of West Nile Virus encephalomyelitis, whereas seizures and head pressing may raise suspicion of an alphaviral encephalitis.

- For an encephalitic horse, differential diagnoses may include Eastern equine encephalitis, Western Equine Encephalitis, Venezuelan equine encephalitis, West Nile Virus, equine protozoal myeloencephalitis (EPM), equine herpesvirus myeloencephalopathy (EHM), Rabies, verminous or bacterial meningoencephalomyelitis, hepatic encephalopathy, and/or leukoencephalomalacia.

- Veterinary practitioners should be aware of the continued emergence of alphavirus and flavivirus infections and the interconnectedness between human and equine health.

DISCLOSURE

There are no commercial or financial conflicts of interest to disclose.

REFERENCES

1. Azar SR, Campos RK, Bergren NA, et al. Epidemic alphaviruses: ecology, emergence and outbreaks. Microorganisms 2020;8(8):1167.
2. Fish D, Tesh RB, Guzman H, et al. Emergence potential of mosquito-borne arboviruses from the Florida Everglades. PLoS One 2021;16(11):e0259419.
3. Anderson JF, Fish D, Armstrong PM, et al. Seasonal dynamics of mosquito-borne viruses in the southwestern florida everglades, 2016, 2017. Am J Trop Med Hyg 2022;106(2):610–22.
4. Colón-González FJ, Sewe MO, Tompkins AM, et al. Projecting the risk of mosquito-borne diseases in a warmer and more populated world: a multi-model, multi-scenario intercomparison modelling study. Lancet Planet Health 2021;5(7):e404–14.
5. Corrin T, Ackford R, Mascarenhas M, et al. Eastern equine encephalitis virus: a scoping review of the global evidence. Vector-Borne Zoonotic Dis 2021;21(5): 305–20.
6. Weaver SC. Host range, amplification and arboviral disease emergence. Arch Virol Suppl 2005;19:33–44.
7. Long MT. West nile virus and equine encephalitis viruses. veterinary clinics of North America: equine practice. Vet Clin North Am Equine Pract 2014;30(3): 523–42.
8. Li L, Lok SM, Yu IM, et al. The flavivirus precursor membrane-envelope protein complex: structure and maturation. Science (1979) 2008;319(5871):1830–2542.
9. Saiz JC, Martín-Acebes MA, Blázquez AB, et al. Pathogenicity and virulence of West Nile virus revisited eight decades after its first isolation. Virulence 2021; 12(1):1145–73.
10. Gould E, Solomon T. Pathogenic flaviviruses. Lancet 2008;371(9611):500–9.

11. Petersen LR, Brault AC, Nasci RS. West Nile Virus: Review of the Literature. JAMA 2013;310(3):308.

12. Kutasi O, Bakonyi T, Lecollinet S, et al. Equine encephalomyelitis outbreak caused by a genetic lineage 2 west nile virus in Hungary. J Vet Intern Med 2011;25(3):586–91.

13. Venter M, Human S, Zaayman D, et al. Lineage 2 West Nile Virus as Cause of Fatal Neurologic Disease in Horses, South Africa. Emerg Infect Dis 2009;15(6): 877–84.

14. Ciota AT. West Nile virus and its vectors. Curr Opin Insect Sci 2017;22:28–36.

15. Turell MJ, O'Guinn ML, Dohm DJ, et al. Vector Competence of North American Mosquitoes (Diptera: Culicidae) for West Nile Virus. J Med Entomol 2001;38(2): 130–4.

16. Hadler J, Nelson R, McCarthy T, et al. West Nile Virus Surveillance in Connecticut in 2000: An Intense Epizootic without High Risk for Severe Human Disease. Emerg Infect Dis 2001;7(4):636–42.

17. Kulasekera VL, Kramer L, Nasci RS, et al. West Nile Virus Infection in Mosquitoes, Birds, Horses, and Humans, Staten Island, New York, 2000. Emerg Infect Dis 2001;7(4):722–5.

18. Komar N, Langevin S, Hinten S, et al. Experimental Infection of North American Birds with the New York 1999 Strain of West Nile Virus. Emerg Infect Dis 2003; 9(3):311–22.

19. Kutzler MA, Bildfell RJ, Gardner-Graff KK, et al. West Nile virus infection in two alpacas. J Am Vet Med Assoc 2004;225(6):921–4.

20. Jacobson ER, Ginn PE, Troutman JM, et al. West Nile virus infection in farmed American alligators (Alligator mississippiensis) in Florida. J Wildl Dis 2005; 41(1):96–106.

21. Yaeger M, Yoon KJ, Schwartz K, et al. West Nile Virus Meningoencephalitis in a Suri Alpaca and Suffolk Ewe. J Vet Diagn Invest 2004;16(1):64–6.

22. Kecskeméti S, Bajmócy E, Á Bacsadi, et al. Encephalitis due to West Nile virus in a sheep. Vet Rec 2007;161(16):568–9.

23. Blackmore CGM, Stark LM, Jeter WC, et al. Surveillance results from the first West Nile virus transmission season in Florida, 2001. Am J Trop Med Hyg 2003;69(2): 141–50.

24. Gingrich JB, Williams GM. Host-feeding patterns of suspected West Nile virus mosquito vectors in Delaware, 2001-2002. J Am Mosq Control Assoc 2005; 21(2):194–200.

25. Gardner IA, Wong SJ, Ferraro GL, et al. Incidence and effects of West Nile virus infection in vaccinated and unvaccinated horses in California. Vet Res 2007; 38(1):109–16.

26. Mackay R, West. Nile and Other Flavivirus Encephalitis. In: Large animal internal medicine. St. Louis, MO: Elsevier; 2020. p. 924–7.

27. Porter MB, Long MT, Getman LM, et al. West Nile Virus encephalomyelitis in horses: 46 cases (2001). J Am Vet Med Assoc 2003;222(9):1241–7.

28. Cantile C, di Guardo G, Eleni C, et al. Clinical and neuropathological features of West Nile virus equine encephalomyelitis in Italy. Equine Vet J 2000;32(1):31–5.

29. Cantile C, del Piero F, di Guardo G, et al. Pathologic and Immunohistochemical Findings in Naturally Occurring West Nile Virus Infection in Horses. Vet Pathol 2001;38(4):414–31.

30. Salazar P, Traub-Dargatz JL, Morley PS, et al. Outcome of equids with clinical signs of West Nile virus infection and factors associated with death. J Am Vet Med Assoc 2004;225(2):267–74.

31. Ward MP, Levy M, Thacker HL, et al. Investigation of an outbreak of encephalomyelitis caused by West Nile virus in 136 horses. J Am Vet Med Assoc 2004; 225(1):84–9.

32. Schuler LA, Khaitsa ML, Dyer NW, et al. Evaluation of an outbreak of West Nile virus infection in horses: 569 cases (2002). J Am Vet Med Assoc 2004;225(7): 1084–9.

33. Porter MB, Long M, Gosche DG, et al. Immunoglobulin M-capture enzyme-linked immunosorbent assay testing of cerebrospinal fluid and serum from horses exposed to west nile virus by vaccination or natural infection. J Vet Intern Med 2004;18(6):866–70.

34. Long MT, Jeter W, Hernandez J, et al. Diagnostic performance of the equine IgM capture ELISA for serodiagnosis of West Nile virus infection. J Vet Intern Med 2006;20(3):608–13.

35. Pennick KE, McKnight CA, Patterson JS, et al. Diagnostic sensitivity and specificity of in situ hybridization and immunohistochemistry for *Eastern equine encephalitis virus* and *West Nile virus* in formalin-fixed, paraffin-embedded brain tissue of horses. J Vet Diagn Invest 2012;24(2):333–8.

36. Delcambre GH, Long MT. Flavivirus Encephalitides. In: Long MT, Sellon D, editors. Equine infectious diseases. 2nd edition. St. Louis: Saunders Elsevier; 2014. p. 217–25.

37. Levasseur A, Arsenault J, Paré J. Surveillance of West Nile virus in horses in Canada: A retrospective study of cases reported to the Canadian Food Inspection Agency from 2003 to 2019. Can Vet J = La revue veterinaire canadienne 2021; 62(5):469–76.

38. Rios LMv, Sheu JJ, Day JF, et al. Environmental risk factors associated with West Nile virus clinical disease in Florida horses. Med Vet Entomol 2009;23(4):357–66.

39. Epp T, Waldner C, West K, et al. Factors associated with West Nile virus disease fatalities in horses. Can Vet J 2007;48(11):1137–45.

40. Chaintoutis SC, Diakakis N, Papanastassopoulou M, et al. Evaluation of cross-protection of a lineage 1 west nile virus inactivated vaccine against natural infections from a virulent lineage 2 strain in horses, under field conditions. Clin Vaccin Immunol 2015;22(9):1040–9.

41. Fehér O, Bakonyi T, Barna M, et al. Serum neutralising antibody titres against a lineage 2 neuroinvasive West Nile Virus strain in response to vaccination with an inactivated lineage 1 vaccine in a European endemic area. Vet Immunol Immunopathol 2020;227:110087.

42. Desanti-Consoli H, Bouillon J, Chapuis RJJ. Equids' Core Vaccines Guidelines in North America: Considerations and Prospective. Vaccines (Basel) 2022; 10(3):398.

43. Heymann D, Heymann D. In: *Control of communicable diseases manual*. 20th edition. Washington DC: American Public Health Association; 2015.

44. From the Centers for Disease Control and Prevention. Possible West Nile virus transmission to an infant through breast-feeding–Michigan. JAMA 2002; 288(16):1976–7.

45. Centers for Disease Control and Prevention (CDC). West Nile virus transmission via organ transplantation and blood transfusion - Louisiana, 2008. MMWR Morb Mortal Wkly Rep 2009;58(45):1263–7.

46. Centers for Disease Control and Prevention (CDC). Update: Investigations of West Nile virus infections in recipients of organ transplantation and blood transfusion. MMWR Morb Mortal Wkly Rep 2002;51(37):833–6.

47. Centers for Disease Control and Prevention (CDC). Investigations of West Nile virus infections in recipients of blood transfusions. MMWR Morb Mortal Wkly Rep 2002;51(43):973–4.
48. Desgraupes S, Hubert M, Gessain A, et al. Mother-to-child transmission of arboviruses during breastfeeding: from epidemiology to cellular mechanisms. Viruses 2021;13(7):1312.
49. Soto RA, McDonald E, Annambhotla P, et al. West Nile virus transmission by solid organ transplantation and considerations for organ donor screening practices, United States. Emerg Infect Dis 2022;28(2):403–6.
50. Mackay R., Alphaviruses, In: Smith B., van Metre D. and Pusterla N., *Large animal internal medicine*, 5th edition., 2020, Elsevier. St. Louis, MO; pp 919–922.
51. Kubes V, Ríos FA. The causative agent of infectious equine encephalomyelitis in Venezuela. Science (1979) 1939;90(2323):20–1.
52. Calisher CH. Medically important arboviruses of the United States and Canada. Clin Microbiol Rev 1994;7(1):89–116.
53. Weaver SC, Winegar R, Manger ID, et al. Alphaviruses: Population genetics and determinants of emergence. Antiviral Res 2012;94(3):242–57.
54. Arrigo NC, Adams AP, Watts DM, et al. Cotton rats and house sparrows as hosts for north and south american strains of eastern equine encephalitis virus. Emerg Infect Dis 2010;16(9):1373–80.
55. Day JF, Stark LM, Zhang JT, et al. Antibodies to arthropod-borne encephalitis viruses in small mammals from southern Florida. J Wildl Dis 1996;32(3):431–6.
56. Morris CD, Srihongse S. An evaluation of the hypothesis of transovarial transmission of eastern equine encephalomyelitis virus by culiseta melanura. Am J Trop Med Hyg 1978;27(6):1246–50.
57. Scott TW, Hildreth SW, Beaty BJ. The distribution and development of eastern equine encephalitis virus in its enzootic mosquito vector, culiseta melanura. Am J Trop Med Hyg 1984;33(2):300–10.
58. Weaver SC, Scott TW, Lorenz LH. Patterns of eastern equine encephalomyelitis virus infection in culiseta melanura (Diptera: Culicidae). J Med Entomol 1990; 27(5):878–91.
59. Reisen WK, Meyer RP, Presser SB, et al. Effect of temperature on the transmission of western equine encephalomyelitis and st. louis encephalitis viruses by culex tarsalis (Diptera: Culicidae). J Med Entomol 1993;30(1):151–60.
60. Armstrong PM, Andreadis TG. Eastern equine encephalitis virus — old enemy, new threat. N Engl J Med 2013;368(18):1670–3.
61. Armstrong PM, Andreadis TG. Ecology and epidemiology of eastern equine encephalitis virus in the northeastern united states: an historical perspective. J Med Entomol 2022;59(1):1–13.
62. Chapman GE, Baylis M, Archer D, et al. The challenges posed by equine arboviruses. Equine Vet J 2018;50(4):436–45.
63. Bedenice D, Bright A, Pedersen DD, et al. Humoral response to an equine encephalitis vaccine in healthy alpacas. J Am Vet Med Assoc 2009;234(4):530–4.
64. Pursell A, Mitchell F, Seibold H. Naturally occurring and experimentally induced eastern encephalomyelitis in calves. J Am Vet Med Assoc 1976;169(10):1101–3.
65. McGee ED, Littleton CH, Mapp JB, et al. Eastern equine encephalomyelitis in an adult cow. Vet Pathol 1992;29(4):361–3.
66. Elvinger F, Baldwin CA, Liggett AD, et al. Prevalence of exposure to eastern equine encephalomyelitis virus in domestic and feral swine in Georgia. J Vet Diagn Invest 1996;8(4):481–4.

67. Bauer RW, Gill MS, Poston RP, et al. Naturally occurring eastern equine encephalitis in a hampshire wether. J Vet Diagn Invest 2005;17(3):281–5.
68. Tate CM, Howerth EW, Stallknecht DE, et al. Eastern equine encephalitis in a free-ranging white-tailed deer (Odocoileus virginianus). J Wildl Dis 2005;41(1):241–5.
69. Mutebi JP, Mathewson AA, Elias SP, et al. Use of Cervid Serosurveys to Monitor Eastern Equine Encephalitis Virus Activity in Northern New England, United States, 2009–2017. J Med Entomol 2022;59(1):49–55.
70. vander Kelen PT, Downs JA, Stark LM, et al. Spatial epidemiology of eastern equine encephalitis in Florida. Int J Health Geographics 2012;11(1):47.
71. Hoff GL, Bigler WJ, Buff EE, et al. Occurrence and distribution of western equine encephalomyelitis in Florida. J Am Vet Med Assoc 1978;172(3):351–2.
72. Sahu SP, Alstad AD, Pedersen DD, et al. Diagnosis of eastern equine encephalomyelitis virus infection in horses by immunoglobulin m and g capture enzyme-linked immunosorbent assay. J Vet Diagn Invest 1994;6(1):34–8.
73. Reisen WK, Lothrop HD, Presser SB, et al. Landscape ecology of arboviruses in southern california: temporal and spatial patterns of vector and virus activity in coachella valley, 1990–1992. J Med Entomol 1995;32(3):255–66.
74. Reisen WK, Lothrop HD, Presser SB, et al. Landscape ecology of arboviruses in southeastern california: temporal and spatial patterns of enzootic activity in imperial valley, 1991–1994. J Med Entomol 1997;34(2):179–88.
75. Burkett-Cadena ND, Day JF, Unnasch TR. Ecology of eastern equine encephalitis virus in the southeastern united states: incriminating vector and host species responsible for virus amplification, persistence, and dispersal. J Med Entomol 2022;59(1):41–8.
76. Carrara AS, Gonzales M, Ferro C, et al. Venezuelan equine encephalitis virus infection of spiny rats. Emerg Infect Dis 2005;11(5):663–9.
77. Carrara AS, Coffey LL, Aguilar Pv, et al. Venezuelan equine encephalitis virus infection of cotton rats. Emerg Infect Dis 2007;13(8):1158–65.
78. Weaver SC, Ferro C, Barrera R, et al. Venezuelan equine encephalitis. Annu Rev Entomol 2004;49:141–74.
79. Zhang M, Fang Y, Brault AC, et al. Variation in western equine encephalomyelitis viral strain growth in mammalian, avian, and mosquito cells fails to explain temporal changes in enzootic and epidemic activity in california. Vector-Borne Zoonotic Dis 2011;11(3):269–75.
80. Reisen WK, Wheeler SS. Surveys for antibodies against mosquitoborne encephalitis viruses in california birds, 1996–2013. Vector-Borne Zoonotic Dis 2016; 16(4):264–82.
81. Robb LL, Hartman DA, Rice L, et al. Continued evidence of decline in the enzootic activity of western equine encephalitis virus in Colorado. J Med Entomol 2019;56(2):584–8.
82. Miller LD, Pearson JE, Muhm RL. A comparison of clinical manifestations and pathology of the equine encephalidites: VEE, WEE, EEE. Proc Annu Meet U S Anim Health Assoc 1973;77:629–31.
83. BYRNE RJ, HETRICK FM, SCANLON JE, et al. Observations on eastern equine encephalitis in Maryland in 1959. J Am Vet Med Assoc 1961;139:661–4.
84. del Piero F, Wilkins PA, Dubovi EJ, et al. Clinical, pathologic, immunohistochemical, and virologic findings of eastern equine encephalomyelitis in two horses. Vet Pathol 2001;38(4):451–6.
85. Long MT, Gibbs EPJ. Equine Alphaviruses. In: Long M, Sellon DC, editors. Equine infectious diseases. 2nd edition. St. Louis: Saunders Elsevier; 2014. p. 210–6.

86. Larsell O, Haring CM, Meyer KF. Histological changes in the central nervous system following equine encephalomyelitis. J Nerv Ment Dis 1935;81(1):80.
87. Gonzalez D, Estrada-Franco JG, Carrara AS, et al. Equine amplification and virulence of subtype ie venezuelan equine encephalitis viruses isolated during the 1993 and 1996 mexican epizootics. Emerg Infect Dis 2003;9(2):162–8.
88. Calisher CH, Mahmud MI, el-Kafrawi AO, et al. Rapid and specific serodiagnosis of western equine encephalitis virus infection in horses. Am J Vet Res 1986;47(6): 1296–9.
89. Cleton NB, van Maanen K, Bergervoet SA, et al. A serological protein microarray for detection of multiple cross-reactive flavivirus infections in horses for veterinary and public health surveillance. Transboundary Emerging Dis 2017;64(6): 1801–12.
90. Gregory CR, Latimer KS, Niagro FD, et al. Detection of eastern equine encephalomyelitis virus rna in formalin-fixed, paraffin-embedded tissues using dna in situ hybridization. J Vet Diagn Invest 1996;8(2):151–5.
91. Patterson JS, Maes RK, Mullaney TP, et al. Immunohistochemical diagnosis of eastern equine encephalomyelitis. J Vet Diagn Invest 1996;8(2):156–60.
92. Linssen B, Kinney RM, Aguilar P, et al. Development of reverse transcription-PCR assays specific for detection of equine encephalitis viruses. J Clin Microbiol 2000;38(4):1527–35.
93. Roehrig JT, Nasci RS, Mitchell CJ, et al. Detection of eastern equine encephalitis virus in infected mosquitoes using a monoclonal antibody-based antigen-capture enzyme-linked immunosorbent assay. Am J Trop Med Hyg 2001;65(3):208–13.
94. Delfraro A, Burgueño A, Morel N, et al. Fatal human case of western equine encephalitis, uruguay. Emerg Infect Dis 2011;17(5):952–4.
95. Tang X, Sedda L, Brown HE. Predicting eastern equine encephalitis spread in North America: An ecological study. Curr Res Parasitol Vector-Borne Dis 2021; 1:100064.
96. Spielman A, Villari P, McDowell M, et al. The economic burden imposed by a residual case of eastern encephalitis. Am J Trop Med Hyg 1995;52(1):8–13.
97. Elias SP, Hoenig DE, Robinson S, et al. An epizootic of eastern equine encephalitis virus, Maine, USA in 2009: outbreak description and entomological studies. Am J Trop Med Hyg 2013;88(1):95–102.

Streptococcus equi Subspecies equi

Ashley G. Boyle, DVM

KEYWORDS

- Strangles • *Streptococcus equi* • Horses • Infectious disease • Lymphatics
- Respiratory

KEY POINTS

- Strangles, caused by the bacteria *Streptococcus equi* subsp *equi*, is a highly contagious disease of equids classically characterized by a high fever and enlarged lymph nodes of the head.
- Diagnostic sampling depends on the stage of the disease.
- The goal of treating strangles is to control transmission and eliminate infection while providing future immunity to the disease. Daily temperature checking and isolation of febrile horses is the key to controlling outbreaks.
- Eradication of this disease will not be possible until *S equi* carriers are cleared.

 Video content accompanies this article at http://www.vetequine.theclinics. com.

INTRODUCTION

Strangles, caused by the gram-positive β-hemolytic, Lancefield group C bacteria *Streptococcus equi* subsp *equi* (*S equi*), is a highly contagious disease of equids. Jordanus Ruffus first described the clinical disease in 1251 Video 1.[1] Strangles is a reportable disease in the United States and many other countries. When unchecked, morbidity can reach 90% to 100% in naïve populations but mortality is typically low.[2–4]

Clinical Signs

Clinical disease is characterized by the sudden onset of fever that can reach as high as 107°F (41.7°C) followed by pharyngitis. Horses typically have an initial serous nasal discharge that develops into a mucopurulent nasal discharge. Abscess formation in submandibular and retropharyngeal lymph nodes develops approximately 1 week after infection (**Fig. 1**). If lymph node enlargement is significant axially, this can result in

Department of Clinical Studies, New Bolton Center, University of Pennsylvania, School of Veterinary Medicine, 382 West Street Road, Kennett Square, PA 19348, USA
E-mail address: boylea@vet.upenn.edu

Vet Clin Equine 39 (2023) 115–131
https://doi.org/10.1016/j.cveq.2022.11.006
0749-0739/23/© 2022 Elsevier Inc. All rights reserved.

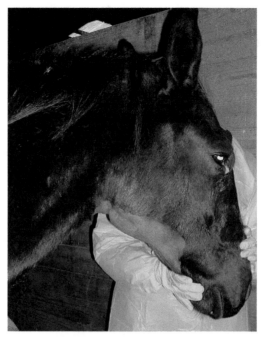

Fig. 1. A horse with classic submandibular lymph node enlargement associated with *S equi* infection. This horse also has ocular discharge that cultured positive for *S equi*.

an obstructed airway and asphyxiation, hence the name "strangles."[5] Often horses will become anorectic and will have an extended head and neck posture. Retropharyngeal lymph nodes may drain into and cause empyema of the guttural pouch (**Fig. 2**). Because this is actually a disease of the lymphatics, other lymph nodes of the body may abscess. Abscesses can form in the parotid, cervical, periorbital, and thoracic inlet regions (see **Fig. 1**) among other sites. Clinical signs usually develop 3 to 14 days after exposure.[1]

Severity of disease depends on the immune status of the patient and the degree of exposure to *S equi* bacterial load. Recently, there has been investigation of a less

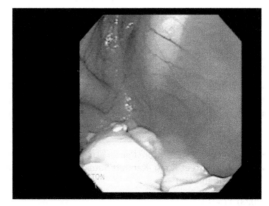

Fig. 2. Endoscopic image of the guttural pouch containing chondroids from a horse that was positive for *S equi*.

virulent strain of *S equi* that infected a crop of naïve weanlings resulting in surprisingly low morbidity and mild clinical signs, highlighting the importance of considering strangles as a differential even if the disease progression is not classic (**Fig. 3**).[6]

Guttural Pouch Empyema and Carrier Status

Many infected horses will have retropharyngeal lymph node drainage into the guttural pouches resulting in guttural pouch empyema. This diagnosis requires endoscopic evaluation or other imaging modalities. Carriers are often defined as horses that are *S equi* positive for greater than 6 weeks.[4,7] These animals may have gross empyema but can be *S equi* positive without it. Prolonged, untreated empyema will result in inspissated purulent material or chondroids. The percentage of carriers per outbreak could be as high as 10% to 42%.[4,8]

Metastatic Disease (Bastard Strangles)

Although often described as an upper respiratory disease, strangles is actually a disease of the lymphatic system. *S equi* can spread hematogenously or lymphatically resulting in metastatic abscessation in 2%[4] to 20%[9] of cases. Common sites of abscessation in metastatic disease include the mesentery, liver, spleen, and kidneys, which can result in peritonitis and clinical signs of colic. Abscessation of the cranial mediastinal lymph nodes can cause tracheal compression and respiratory distress. Abscessation within the brain has been documented.[10] In addition, aspiration of mucopurulent discharge can cause pneumonia. The presence of metastatic abscessation can increase the mortality rate to as high as 62% if not aggressively treated.[11,12]

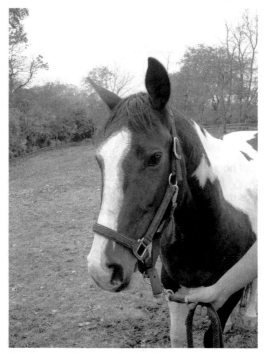

Fig. 3. A *S equi*–positive horse with atypical strangles presentation. This horse only had mild mucopurulent discharge and a fever.

Purpura Hemorrhagica

Purpura hemorrhagica is a type III hypersensitivity that results in an aseptic necrotizing vasculitis that can occur in mature horses after repeated natural exposure to S equi infection or after S equi vaccination of horses that have had strangles. The actual incidence of this reaction is unknown. In some cases, antigen–antibody complexes affect other sites, including the gastrointestinal tract, muscles, lungs, myocardium, and kidneys. Clinical signs range from mild to life-threatening, including pitting edema of the head, trunk, and distal limbs, as well as petechiae and ecchymoses.[13,14]

Myositis

Three significant myopathies have been documented after exposure to S equi. These include muscle infarctions, rhabdomyolysis with acute myonecrosis, and rhabdomyolysis with progressive atrophy.[15–17] In Quarter Horses, a missense mutation in MYH1 has been associated with rhabdomyolysis with progressive atrophy, which is a type of immune-mediated myositis.[18]

Pathogenesis

S equi enters through the mouth or nose and attaches to cells in the crypts of the lingual and palatine tonsils as well as the epithelium of the pharyngeal and tubal tonsils. The organism is difficult to detect on the mucosal surface resulting in negative culture of nasal and nasopharyngeal samples during early infection. Translocation occurs in a few hours to the mandibular and retropharyngeal lymph nodes.[19]

Polymorphonuclear neutrophils are attracted by complement-derived chemotactic factors resulting in visible abscessation of the lymph node 3 to 5 days after entry.[20] The hyaluronic acid capsule, antiphagocytic SeM protein, and Mac protein aid in the organism's evasion of phagocytosis.[21]

Shedding

Nasal shedding of S equi usually begins 1 to 2 days after onset of fever. This important fact makes it possible to isolate any horses with a new fever before they start shedding. Many animals shed for approximately 3 weeks but others can shed for at least 6 weeks after purulent discharges have stopped. Persistent guttural pouch infection may result in intermittent shedding for years.[22–24]

Immunity

Approximately 75% of horses develop a waning immunity to strangles that lasts about 5 years after recovery from the disease.[25–27] It has been shown that serologic response to disease is decreased in horses that have been treated with antibiotics,[4,28] suggesting that immunity is not as strong in these animals and they may be susceptible to reinfection. Older horses with residual immunity have limited susceptibility and develop a mild form of strangles but shed virulent S equi that will produce severe disease in more susceptible, often younger horses.[1] Foals obtain maternal antibodies via colostrum and milk that coat the upper respiratory and oral mucosa and are usually resistant to S equi infection until weaning.[29]

Diagnosis

Early definitive diagnosis is essential for containing this highly infectious pathogen. Sampling may be unsuccessful during the incubation and early clinical phases because S equi is normally not present on the mucosa until at least 24 to 48 hours after the onset of fever.[19,30] Monitoring temperatures daily and isolating horses that are febrile, or have an increase in their normal temperature pattern, is the key to control the spread of infection.

Cytology and Hematology

Cytologic evaluation reveals gram-positive extracellular cocci in long chains, supporting a general diagnosis of a β-hemolytic streptococcus organism. Common hematologic findings of horses with *S equi* are nonspecific: an increase in inflammatory proteins such as serum amyloid A and fibrinogen, a neutrophilic leukocytosis, and mild anemia.[4,31] Horses with metastatic disease are likely to have a more significant anemia due to chronic disease.[11] Horses with purpura hemorrhagica can have alterations in their coagulation profiles.[13]

Samples

Samples can be obtained through aspirate of mature lymph nodes, a nasopharyngeal swab, a nasopharyngeal wash, or a guttural pouch wash. A comparison of *S equi* sample type is found in **Table 1**.[1]

Culture

Culture is the preferred method on aspirates of mature abscesses and is inexpensive, sensitive, and accurate for samples that have large numbers of bacteria, such as those collected from animals with obvious disease. It takes a minimum of 24 hours to obtain

Table 1
Comparison of sample type for the diagnosis of *Streptococcus equi*

S equi Sample	Pros	Cons
Aspirate of mature abscessed lymph node	High yield of bacterial organisms	Requires this stage of disease
Moistened rostral nasal swab[a]	Ease of sampling	Animal needs to have active mucopurulent discharge
Moistened nasopharyngeal swab[a]	Ease of sampling	False negatives possible in early febrile state (not shedding yet) False negatives possible due to intermittent shedding from guttural pouch
Nasopharyngeal wash	Ease of sampling	False negatives possible in early febrile state (not shedding yet)
	Sampling more surface area Was found to be more sensitive than nasopharyngeal swab	False negatives possible due to intermittent shedding from guttural pouch
Guttural pouch lavage	Best for detection of carrier animals	Special equipment needed
	Can increase sensitivity by combining guttural pouch lavage with nasopharyngeal wash by collecting at the nose	Experience entering the guttural pouch More time consuming False negative if lymph nodes have not yet ruptured into the pouch

[a] Synthetic microfiber flocked swabs have not shown increased detection rates over traditional rayon or cotton swabs.

Boyle AG, Timoney JF, Newton JR, et al. Streptococcus equi Infections in Horses: Guidelines for Treatment, Control, and Prevention of Strangles-Revised Consensus Statement. J Vet Intern Med. 2018 Mar;32(2):633-647.

results. Up to 40% of samples can be falsely negative on culture, especially in patients sampled too early in the course of disease or during convalescence.[30]

Polymerase chain reaction

Multiple gene targets are available for the detection of *S equi* through quantitative polymerase chain reaction (qPCR), and this technique has been shown to be more sensitive than culture as a diagnostic tool.[30,32,33] Nasopharyngeal washes are preferable to nasopharyngeal swabs due to a larger sampling area[30] but guttural pouch sampling is 50 times more likely to detect carrier animals.[34] Combined guttural pouch and nasopharyngeal sampling (collecting the sample from the guttural pouch at the nose) may increase the positive yield even further as a positive nasopharynx and negative guttural pouch is rare but possible.[35] Absence of obvious guttural pouch pathologic condition on endoscopic evaluation combined with negative guttural pouch lavage qPCR is recommended to remove a horse from quarantine.[1] The endoscope should be sterilized following and between sampling of suspect horses. Three, consecutive nasopharyngeal washes have been shown to accurately identify carrier animals, although, in this study, there was a delay in endoscopy by a few months.[36]

There has been much controversy over whether a qPCR-positive, culture-negative animal is still infectious. Two studies provide evidence that suggest that these animals should be considered a threat to naïve populations. Pringle and colleagues[35] showed that *S equi* PCR–positive, culture-negative horses can become culture positive again. Morris and colleagues[37] used genomic testing to reveal that an outbreak occurred of the same strain of *S equi* when only negative cultures of the guttural pouch samples were used to clear horses to reenter the herd.

Serology

Two different serology tests are available throughout the world. The purpose of these tests depends on the test and the setting in which it is used.

SeM Protein

Serology detecting antibody titers to SeM surface protein is available in the United States and Europe. It can be used for the following purposes:

1. Detection of recent infection evidenced by a 4-fold or greater increase in paired titers taken 10 days apart. It typically peaks at 5 weeks after infection and can remain high for at least 6 months.
2. Support a diagnosis of purpura hemorrhagica or metastatic abscessation (titer $\geq$1:12,800).[1]
3. Safety of vaccination. It has been suggested that horses with high serum SeM-specific antibody titers ($\geq$1:3200) may be predisposed to developing purpura hemorrhagica when vaccinated against *S equi*.[1] A 2009 study reported safely vaccinating horses with SeM titers of 1:1600[13] or less with the Pinnacle I.N. (Zoetis, Parsipanny, NJ) vaccine.[38] A 2017 study suggested that horses should be tested with the SeM serology for 1 year after a strangles outbreak to determine when it is safe to vaccinate.[39] Not all high titers ($\geq$1:12,800) mean there are complications. Delph and colleagues[40] showed that SeM antibody titers can be increased after infection without complications.

Combined Antigen A (SEQ_2190 N-Terminal Fragment) and Antigen C (SeM N-Terminal Fragment)

This combined indirect enzyme-linked immunosorbent assay (iELISA) detects 2 surface antigens: Antigen A (SEQ_2190 N-Terminal Fragment) and Antigen C (SeM

N-Terminal Fragment). It has similar sensitivity but greater specificity when compared with the whole SeM antibody titer.[41] It is currently available in Europe, Australia, and Dubai. This iELISA is recommended

1. To identify horses with strangles exposure as recent as 2 weeks previously and
2. To identify animals without clinical signs that may be carrying *S equi* for the purposes of isolation and further evaluation through endoscopic guttural pouch examination.[8,41,42]

Most current vaccines cross react with both serology tests.[43,44] This warrants the need for vaccines that are differentiate infected from vaccinated animals (DIVA) to enable the identification of recently infected horses from already vaccinated animals through serology. A recent study showed a failure to identify subclinical *S equi* carriers using the combined Antigen A and C iELISA,[45] which has resulted in the recommendation of using the test within 6 months of an outbreak (Andrew Waller, Intervacc AB, personal communication). Neither SeM ELISA nor the combined iELISA confirm empyema or carrier status.[41,42,46]

Outbreak Control

Sources of infection
Besides the obviously ill horses that are known to be shedding *S equi*, healthy appearing horses can also potentially shed *S equi*. When brought into a naïve population, these horses can be the source of infection. Examples include horses that are incubating the disease and go on to develop clinical signs, horses that are recovering from recent disease but that continue to harbor the organism after full clinical recovery for some weeks, and horses that are fully recovered from the disease but continue to be potentially infectious for prolonged periods through periodic shedding of *S equi* (carriers).[1] Definitive determination of carrier status requires endoscopic examination of the guttural pouches as well as PCR testing of guttural pouch lavage fluid.[1,47] Many farms with repeated infections have resorted to screening for infection through a single endoscopic evaluation and PCR testing of guttural pouch lavage.[47]

Table 2 shows the aims of infection control and the measures that can be taken to meet those aims.[1,48,49]

Treatment
The goal of treating strangles is to control transmission and eliminate infection while providing future immunity to the disease. Antibiotic treatment has been shown to reduce the serologic response to disease, therefore affecting immunity in these animals.[4,28] Appropriate treatment of horses with strangles usually depends on the stage and severity of the disease.[50]

Early acute phase
Treatment with antibiotics in the early acute phase with fever and depression only may be curative and may prevent focal abscessation and shedding. Antibiotics have adequate access to the bacteria if abscesses have not formed. This immediate treatment of horses with fever only could be effective at controlling outbreaks, although the disadvantages of treatment (lack of immunity) should be considered.[1]

Lymph node abscessation
Uncomplicated cases with lymph node abscessation should be treated with supportive care in order to provide lasting immunity. Affected horses should be isolated where they can stay dry and fed moist, palatable food. Nonsteroidal anti-inflammatory drugs (NSAIDs) should be used judiciously to decrease swelling, reduce fever, and promote

Table 2
Aims and measures used to control transmission of *Streptococcus equi* on affected premises

Aim	Measure
1. To prevent the spread of *S equi* infection to horses on other premises and to new arrivals on the affected premises	Quarantine new arrivals for 3 wk. Additional screening for subclinical carriers by guttural pouch endoscopy, culture, and qPCR testing should be part of any screening program. Stop all movement of horses on and off the affected premises immediately and until further notice
	Horses with strangles and their contacts should be maintained in well-demarcated "dirty" (ie, *S equi*–positive) quarantine areas
	Clustering of cases in groups should allow parts of the premises to allocated as "dirty" (red), "exposed" (amber), and "clean" (green) areas
	Perform twice-daily monitoring of rectal temperatures of the amber and green group to identify temperature increases in horses early and move them to the red area before the start of shedding
2. To establish whether convalescing horses are infectious at least 3 wk after clinical recovery	Testing horses that have been treated with antibiotics should not commence before 3 wk after the cessation of antibiotic treatment. If nasal discharge persists longer than 2 wk, guttural pouch examination is indicated to identify horses that may have empyema and require additional treatment. 1 endoscopically guided guttural pouch lavage qPCR on cases and their contacts to screen for carriers provides increased efficiency and sensitivity over 3 nasopharyngeal washes during 3 wk. All equipment must be disinfected among horses when sampling multiples on a farm
	Horses are considered safe to move out of isolation from the absence of obvious guttural pouch pathologic condition in conjunction with negative guttural pouch lavage qPCR results
3. To eliminate *S equi* infection from the guttural pouches	Remove pathologic condition through a combination of flushing and aspiration with saline, and remove chondroids using endoscopically guided instruments
	Perform topical and systemic administration of antimicrobials to eliminate *S equi* infection
	A minimum of 3 wk should pass before retesting a treated, previously positive guttural pouch via qPCR
4. To prevent indirect cross-infection by *S equi* from horses in the "dirty" area to those in the "clean" area of the premises	Personnel should use dedicated protective clothing when dealing with infectious animals and should not deal simultaneously with susceptible animals
	If this is unavoidable, infectious horses should be dealt with *after* susceptible animals
	Strict hygiene measures are introduced, including provision of dedicated clothing and equipment for each area and disinfection facilities for personnel and use of thorough stable cleaning and disinfection methods
	When cost is not a factor, consideration should be given to destruction of the dedicated equipment after eradication of the infection

(continued on next page)

Table 2 *(continued)*	
Aim	Measure
	After removal of organic material from stables, all surfaces should be cleaned first with detergent and then be thoroughly soaked in an appropriate liquid disinfectant (bleach, phenols, quaternary ammonium compounds) and allowed to dry
	Manure and waste feed from infectious animals should be composted (disinfected by heat) in an isolated location
	Pastures used to hold infectious animals should be rested for 4 wk
	Care should be taken to clean and disinfect water troughs at least once daily during an outbreak
	Horse vans should be cleaned with detergent and then disinfected after each use

Adapted from Boyle, AG. Streptococcus equi subsp. equi infection (Strangles). In: Smith NP, Van Metre DC, Pusterla N, editors. Large Animal Internal Medicine. 6th edition. St. Louis: Elsevier; 2020. P. 559-564; with permission. (Box 31-9 in original).

eating. Maturation of abscesses can be promoted with the use of hot compresses or topical 20% ichthammol. Once mature, external abscesses should be lanced to allow drainage, followed by daily lavage using dilute ("weak tea" colored) povidone iodine solution.

If the horse is nonresponsive to supportive therapy and NSAIDs and continues to have fevers, anorexia, or any signs of dyspnea, antibiotic therapy is recommended. Rarely, severe cases may require intensive supportive therapy, including IV fluids, feeding by nasogastric tube, and tracheostomy.

Antibiotic choice

Penicillin G (procaine penicillin [22,000–44,000 IU/kg IM q12 h] or aqueous potassium penicillin [22,000–44,000 IU/kg IV q6 h]) is considered the drug of choice for the treatment of nonpneumococcal streptococcal disease. Recently, *S equi* samples resistant to penicillin have been identified.[51] In addition, *S equi* samples with altered phenotype have been described that had mutations to pbp2x, which has been previously associated with penicillin resistance in *Streptococcus pneumoniae*.[37] These 2 facts warrant monitoring for resistance going forward and submitting samples for culture and sensitivity. Other agents for therapy include cephalosporins[52] but should be reserved for cases indicated by culture or for patients that are significantly noncompliant to treatment with penicillin. Oral options include chloramphenicol and trimethoprim-sulfadiazine. Trimethoprim-sulfadiazine treatment failure has been seen in the closely related *Streptococcus equi* subsp *zooepidemicus*,[53] although a recent study showed in vitro susceptibility in 100% of *S equi* isolates recovered in Colombia.[54]

Treatment of Carriers/Empyema

Elimination of guttural pouch empyema requires repeated lavage using polyethylene tubing through an endoscope, through a Chamber's catheter, or an indwelling Foley catheter. A 20% solution of acetylcysteine in buffered saline can be useful to break up disulfide bonds in mucoproteins.[55] Some thick empyema and chondroids are particularly difficult to remove, requiring manual removal with endoscopic equipment, such as a memory helical polyp retrieval basket, or surgical removal. (Video 1)

Successful elimination of *S equi* in these carriers requires local treatment of the guttural pouch with penicillin after the removal of the material within the guttural pouch in addition to systemic treatment with procaine penicillin or potassium penicillin for 7 to 10 days.[47,56,57] The use of reverse thermodynamic gel (liquid when cool and solid when warm) has been used for local delivery of antibiotics to treat chronic shedders.[58]

Treatment of Bastard Strangles

If possible, culture and sensitivity from the affected body cavity provides the direction for the appropriate antibiotic treatment, which has included penicillin, ceftiofur, chloramphenicol, and doxycycline.[59] In one study, an average of 2.5 months of antibiotic treatment was needed for resolution.[11] Monitoring of fibrinogen can assist in determining the duration of treatment with cessation of treatment after normalization of fibrinogen levels. Some horses have been treated via surgical drainage along with systemic antibiotics.[12,59]

Treatment of Purpura Hemorrhagica

In addition to prolonged treatment with penicillin, cases of purpura hemorrhagica also require the use of systemic corticosteroids (dexamethasone, 0.1–0.2 mg/kg IV or IM q12–24 h; prednisolone, 0.5–1 mg/kg PO q24 h) for an average of 3 weeks to reduce systemic vasculitis.[13]

Vaccination

Vaccines should be administered only to healthy nonfebrile animals free of nasal discharge. Although controversial, vaccination is not recommended during an outbreak. Christmann and colleagues[52] showed a high rate of purpura hemorrhagic when attenuated live intranasal vaccine (Pinnacle I.N. [Zoetis, Parsipanny, N.J.]) was used on a large standardbred farm during an outbreak.

Extract Vaccines

Extract vaccines (Strepvax II [Boehringer Ingelheim Vetmedica, Inc., St. Joseph, Mo.]) are labeled to "aid in the reduction of disease" and to be given intramuscularly (preferably in the hindquarters). The vaccine elicits serum antibody responses 7 to 10 days later. Naive horses and foals require a schedule of 3 doses at an interval of 3 weeks with a booster given once annually. Pregnant mares may be boostered a month before expected date of foaling.[60] Extract vaccines have been associated with cases of purpura hemorrhagica.[13]

Attenuated Live Intranasal Vaccine

Attenuated live vaccine (Pinnacle I.N. [Zoetis, Parsipanny, N.J.]) is given intranasally in a schedule of 2 doses at 2-week to 3-week intervals and is labeled to "aid in the prevention of disease." Annual booster doses are recommended. Careful handling of live vaccine is essential to prevent inadvertent injection intramuscularly either through the vaccine directly or contamination of other vaccines given at the same time. A temporary pharyngitis is possible secondary to administration of this vaccine.[61] Although labeled for animals 9 months and older, further studies suggest that it not be recommended in horses aged less than 1 year due to the possible development of vaccine-associated clinical disease.[62,63] As mentioned above, attenuated live vaccine has also been associated with cases of purpura hemorrhagica.[52]

Recombinant Fusion Protein Vaccine

Recent experimental trials in Europe have evaluated the use of recombinant multicomponent subunit vaccines (Strangvac [Intervacc, AB Sweden]). At the time of this writing, it is approved for use in Sweden and awaiting approval for use in other European countries and the United Kingdom. This vaccine has DIVA capabilities that would enable its use with serology.[64,65]

Epidemiology

Prevalence

Strangles is found throughout the world except in Iceland. There are a few studies examining the prevalence of strangles in the equine population around the world but interpretation varies based on type of testing (serology, culture, and PCR), population sampled (laboratory samples vs general equine population), and the anatomical site sampled (rostral nasal passage vs guttural pouch). Seroprevalence, using the combined iELISA, has been shown to be around 10% in South Africa and Israel.[66,67] Using rostral nasal swabs, 2.3% prevalence of disease was found in healthy horses in Brazil,[68] whereas 15.3% of horses in a general Colombian population were culture positive on guttural pouch swabs.[54] Seven United Kingdom laboratories reported 1617 positive strangles diagnoses between January 1, 2015 and December 31, 2019.[69]

Environmental Persistence of Streptococcus equi

Historically, Jorm and colleagues[70] looked at the length of survival on glass (48 days) and wood (63 days) in the laboratory setting. *S equi* was cultured from swabs for only 3 days from fence line and rubber when examined in a simulated outdoor setting. Full sunlight decreased survival to a day or less. The presence of mucous increased the chance of a positive culture greater than 1 day compared with less than one day.[71] When examining multiple types of surfaces, bacterial viability was shown to be enhanced by a wet environment and colder weather. *S equi* survived up to 9 days in wet sites and 2 days in dry sites in the summer but survived up to 34 days in wet sites and 13 days in dry sites in the winter.[72] A small percentage (0.54%) of face flies collected from a farm with a strangles outbreak were found to be positive for *S equi* through qPCR, highlighting the need to institute fly control to decrease the chance of transmission.[73]

Twitches and Endoscopes

Researchers recommend the use of sedatives instead of twitches when working with *S equi*–positive horses. Sections of twitch rope were still culture positive even after cleaning with a surfactant-based cleaner; a disinfection step was necessary to make them culture negative. Only sodium hypochlorite eliminated DNA resulting in a negative PCR. Endoscopes used to sample chronic *S equi* carriers were found to be culture negative but 1 out of 14 was still positive for DNA after aggressive cleaning and disinfection. The best success was using a cleaning system with a brush.[74]

Zoonosis

S equi infection can be a zoonotic disease for people with immunosuppression. A recent case report described *S equi* meningitis and a subdural abscess in a 13-year-old child with lupus that was contracted from a sick pony.[75]

FUTURE DIRECTIONS

Different point-of-care diagnostic technologies are becoming available. A PCR that could be run in clinic is now available that has a sensitivity of 84% and specificity of 89% from rostral nasal swabs. It is best used for index cases, not detecting carriers that have a low amount of DNA in their samples.[76] Loop-mediated amplification technology has also been used to detect strangles in convalescent carriers with good success compared with a qPCR.[77] This technology could be used on farm, although this is currently not commercially available. Recent studies have looked at DNA viability testing in combination with PCR with success but it is known that bacteria can become nonviable in transit running the risk of misidentifying potential infectious bacteria as noninfectious.[78,79]

Genomic studies have become a large body of work in the recent research on *S equi*. There is genomic evidence that strangles strains are similar throughout the world, providing proof that the disease has been carried across the world through global equine travel. This is an argument for it to be listed as a World Organization for Animal Health (formerly the Office International des Epizooties) reportable disease.[37,80] There was no genomic difference between the *S equi* samples from acute and carrier cases of strangles leading the authors to suggest that future research needs to examine the host response instead.[7]

SUMMARY

With the combination of new vaccines, improved diagnostics, future investigations into the host response, and identifying carriers, the future looks brighter for the control of this highly contagious disease.

CLINICS CARE POINTS

- Water troughs are a common source of infection.
- Separating horses into red ("dirty"), amber ("in contacts"), and green ("clean") groups will help control infections.
- If a horse has nasal discharge for longer than two weeks, guttural pouch endoscopy is recommended.

DISCLOSURE

Dr A.G. Boyle currently has a grant from Boehringer Ingelheim, United States supporting research on strangles.

SUPPLEMENTARY DATA

Supplementary data related to this article can be found online at https://doi.org/10.1016/j.cveq.2022.11.006.

REFERENCES

1. Boyle AG, Timoney JF, Newton JR, et al. Streptococcus equi infections in horses: guidelines for treatment, control, and prevention of strangles-revised consensus statement. J Vet Intern Med 2018;32(2):633–47.

2. George JL, Reif JS, Shiedeler RK, et al. Identification of carriers of Streptococcus equi in a naturally infected herd. J Am Vet Med Assoc 1983;183:8–84.

3. Sweeney CR, Benson CE, Whitlock RH, et al. Description of an epizootic and persistence of Streptococcus equi infections in horses. J Am Vet Med Assoc 1989;194:1281–5.

4. Duffee LR, Stefanovski D, Boston RC, et al. Predictor variables for and complications associated with Streptococcus equi subsp equi infection in horses. J Am Vet Med Assoc 2015;247:1161–8.

5. Waller AS. New perspectives for the diagnosis, control, treatment, and prevention of strangles in horses. Vet Clin North Am Equine Pract 2014;30:591–607.

6. Tscheschlok L, Venner M, Steward K, et al. Decreased clinical severity of strangles in weanlings associated with restricted seroconversion to optimized streptococcus equi ssp equi assays. J Vet Intern Med 2018;32:459–64.

7. Morris ERA, Boyle AG, Riihimäki M, et al. Differences in the genome, methylome, and transcriptome do not differentiate isolates of Streptococcus equi subsp. equi from horses with acute clinical signs from isolates of inapparent carriers. PLoS One 2021;16:e0252804.

8. Pringle J, Venner M, Tscheschlok L, et al. Markers of long term silent carriers of Streptococcus equi ssp. equi in horses. J Vet Intern Med 2020;34:2751–7.

9. Sweeney CR, Whitlock RH, Meirs DA, et al. Complications associated with Streptococcus equi infection on a horse farm. J Am Vet Med Assoc 1987;191:1446–8.

10. Finno C, Pusterla N, Aleman M, et al. Streptococcus equi meningoencephalomyelitis in a foal. J Am Vet Med Assoc 2006;229:721–4.

11. Pusterla N, Whitcomb MB, Wilson WD. Internal abdominal abscesses caused by Streptococcus equi subspecies equi in 10 horses in California between 1989 and 2004. Vet Rec 2007;160:589.

12. Mair TS, Sherlock CE. Surgical drainage and post operative lavage of large abdominal abscesses in six mature horses. Equine Vet J Suppl 2011;39:123.

13. Pusterla N, Watson JL, Affolter VK, et al. Purpura haemorrhagica in 53 horses. Vet Rec 2003;153:118–21.

14. Galán JE, Timoney JF. Immune complexes in purpura hemorrhagica of the horse contain IgA and M antigen of Streptococcus equi. J Immunol 1985;135:3134–7.

15. Kaese HJ, Valberg SJ, Hayden DW, et al. Infarctive purpura hemorrhagica in five horses. J Am Vet Med Assoc 2005;226:1893–8.

16. Sponseller BT, Valberg SJ, Tennent-Brown B, et al. Severe acute rhabdomyolysis in 4 horses associated with Streptococcus equi subspecies equi infection. J Am Vet Med Assoc 2005;227:1800–7.

17. Hunyadi L, Sundman EA, Kass PH, et al. Clinical Implications and Hospital Outcome of Immune-Mediated Myositis in Horses. J Vet Intern Med 2017;31:170–5.

18. Finno CJ, Gianino G, Perumbakkam S, et al. A missense mutation in MYH1 is associated with susceptibility to immune-mediated myositis in Quarter Horses. Skelet Muscle 2018;8:7.

19. Timoney JF, Kumar P. Early pathogenesis of equine Streptococcus equi infection(strangles) Equine. Vet J 2008;40:637–42.

20. Mukhtar MM, Timoney JF. Chemotactic response of equine polymorphonuclear leucocytes to Streptococcus equi. Res Vet Sci 1988;45:225–9.

21. Timoney JF, Suther P, Velineni S, Artiushin C. The antiphagocytic activity of SeM OF Streptococcus equi requires capsule. J Equine Sci 2014;25:53–6.

22. Chanter N, Newton JR, Wood JLN, et al. Detection of strangles carriers. Vet Rec 1998;142:496.

23. Newton JR, Wood JLN, Dunn KA, et al. Naturally occurring persistent and asymptomatic infection of the guttural pouches of horses with Streptococcus equi. Vet Rec 1997;140:84–90.

24. Newton JR, Wood JLN, Chanter N. Strangles: long term carriage of Streptococcus equi in horses. Equine Vet Ed 1997;9:98–102.

25. Todd TG. Strangles J Comp Path Therap 1910;23:212–29.

26. Hamlen HJ, Timoney JF, Bell RJ. Epidemiologic and immunologic characteristics of Streptococcus equi infection in foals. J Am Vet Med Assoc 1994;204:768–75.

27. Timoney JF, Qin A, Muthupalani S, et al. Vaccine potential of novel surface exposed and secreted proteins of Streptococcus equi. Vaccine 2007;25:5583–90.

28. Pringle J, Storm E, Waller A, et al. Influence of penicillin treatment of horses with strangles on seropositivity to Streptococcus equi ssp. equi-specific antibodies. J Vet Intern Med 2020;34:294–9.

29. Galan JE, Timoney JF, Lengemann FW. Passive transfer of mucosal antibody to Streptococcus equi in the foal. Infect Immun 1986;54:202–6.

30. Lindahl S, Baverud V, Egenvall A, et al. Comparison of Sampling Sites and Laboratory Diagnostic Tests for S equi subsp. equi in Horses from Confirmed Strangles Outbreaks. J Vet Intern Med 2013;27:542–7.

31. Jerele S, Davis E, Mapes S, et al. Survey of Serum Amyloid A and Bacterial and Viral Frequency Using qPCR Levels in Recently Captured Feral Donkeys from Death Valley National Park (California). Animals 2020;10:1086.

32. Boyle AG, Boston RC, O'Shea K, et al. Optimization of an in vitro assay to detect Streptococcus equi subsp. equi. Vet Microbiol 2012;159:406.

33. Boyle AG, Rankin SC, Duffee L, et al. S equi detection PCR assay for equine nasopharyngeal and guttural pouch wash samples. J Vet Intern Med 2016;30:276–81.

34. Boyle AG, Stefanovski D, Rankin SC. Determining optimal sampling site for Streptococcus equi subsp equi carriers using loop-mediated isothermal amplification. BMC Vet Res 2017;13:75.

35. Pringle J, Venner M, Tscheschlok L, et al. Long term silent carriers of Streptococcus equi ssp. equi following strangles; carrier detection related to sampling site of collection and culture versus qPCR. Vet J 2019;246:66–70.

36. Pringle J, Aspán A, Riihimäki M. Repeated nasopharyngeal lavage predicts freedom from silent carriage of Streptococcus equi after a strangles outbreak. J Vet Intern Med 2022;36:787–91.

37. Morris ERA, Hillhouse AE, Konganti K, et al. Comparison of whole genome sequences of Streptococcus equi subsp. equi from an outbreak in Texas with isolates from within the region, Kentucky, USA, and other countries. Vet Microbiol 2020;243:108638.

38. Boyle AG, Sweeney CR, Kristula M, et al. Factors associated with likelihood of horses having a high serum Streptococcus equi SeM-specific antibody titer. J Am Vet Med Assoc 2009;235:973.

39. Boyle AG, Smith MA, Boston RC, et al. SeM titers after natural outbreaks of Streptococcus equi equi in horses: a case-control study. J Am Vet Med Assoc 2017;250:1432–9.

40. Delph KM, Beard LA, Trimble AC, et al. Strangles, convalescent Streptococcus equi subspecies equi M antibody titers, and presence of complications. J Vet Intern Med 2019;33:275–9.

41. Robinson C, Steward KF, Potts N, et al. Combining two serological assays optimises sensitivity and specificity for the identification of Streptococcus equi subsp. equi exposure. Vet J 2013;197:188–91.

42. Knowles EJ, Mair TS, Butcher N, et al. Use of a novel serological test for exposure to Streptococcus equi subspecies equi in hospitalised horses. Vet Rec 2010; 166:294.

43. Boyle AG, Mitchell C, Stefanovski D, et al. Horses vaccinated with live attenuated intranasal strangles vaccine seroconvert to SEQ2190 and SeM. Equine Vet J 2022;54:299–305.

44. El-Hage CM, Bannai H, Wiethoelter AK, et al. Serological responses of Australian horses using a commercial duplex indirect ELISA following vaccination against strangles. Aust Vet J 2019;97:220–4.

45. Durham AE, Kemp-Symonds J. Failure of serological testing for antigens A and C of Streptococcus equi subspecies equi to identify guttural pouch carriers. Equine Vet J 2021;53:38–43.

46. Davidson A, Traub-Dargatz JL, Magnuson R, et al. Lack of correlation between antibody titers to fibrinogen-binding protein of Streptococcus equi and persistent carriers of strangles. J Vet Diagn Invest 2008;20:457.

47. Newton JR, Verheyen K, Talbot NC, et al. Control of strangles outbreaks by isolation of guttural pouch carriers identified using PCR and culture of Streptococcus equi. Equine Vet J 2000;32:515.

48. Boyle AG. Strangles and its complications. Eq Vet Educ 2017;29:149–57.

49. Boyle AG. Streptococcus equi subsp. equi infection (Strangles). In: Smith NP, Van Metre DC, Pusterla N, editors. Large animal internal medicine. 6th edition. St. Louis: Elsevier; 2020. p. 559–64.

50. Ramey D. Does early antibiotic use in horses with "strangles" cause metastatic Streptococcus equi bacterial infections? Equine Vet Educ 2007;19:14.

51. Fonesca JD, Mavrides DE, Morgan AL, et al. Antibiotic resistance in bacteria associated with equine respiratory disease in the United Kingdom. Vet Rec 2020;187:189.

52. Christmann U, Pink C. Lessons learned from a strangles outbreak on a large Standardbred farm. Eq Vet Educ 2017;29:138–43.

53. Ensink JM, Bosch G, Van Duijkeren E. Clinical efficacy of prophylactic administration of trimethoprim/sulfadiazine in a Streptococcus equi subsp. zooepidemicus infection model in ponies. J Vet Pharmacol Ther 2005;28:45.

54. Jaramillo-Morales C, Gomez DE, Renaud D, et al. Streptococcus equi culture prevalence, associated risk factors and antimicrobial susceptibility in a horse population from Colombia. J Equine Vet Sci 2022;111:103890.

55. Plumb DC. Acetylcysteine. In: Plumbs veterinary drug handbook. 9 th edition. Hoboken: Wiley-Blackwell; 2018.

56. Verheyen K, Newton JR, Talbot NC, et al. Elimination of guttural pouch infection and inflammation in asymptomatic carriers of Streptococcus equi. Equine Vet J 2000;32:527–32.

57. Waller A, Robinson C, Newton JR. Further thoughts on the eradication of strangles in equids. J Am Vet Med Assoc 2007;231:1335.

58. Bowen M. Use of a reverse thermodynamic gel to manage chronic shedding in equine strangles. Vet Evid 2017;2:109.

59. Broux B, Bergen T van, Schauvliege S, et al. Successful surgical debridement of a cerebral Streptococcus equi equi abscess by parietal bone flap craniotomy in a 2-month-old Warmblood foal. Equine Vet Education 2019;31:e58–62.

60. Strepvax II. Available at: https://www.bi-vetmedica.com/species/equine/products/strepvax.html#tabs-1-2. Accessed June 29, 2022.

61. Pinnacle IN. Available at: https://www2.zoetisus.com/products/equine/pinnacle-in. Accessed June 29, 2022.

62. Borst LB, Patterson SK, Lanka S, et al. Evaluation of a commercially available modified-live Streptococcus equi subsp equi vaccine in ponies. Am J Vet Res 2011;72:1130–8.

63. Cursons R, Patty O, Steward KF, et al. Strangles in horses can be caused by vaccination with Pinnacle I. N Vaccin 2015 Jul 9;33:3440–3.

64. Robinson C, Frykberg L, Flock M, et al. Strangvac: a recombinant fusion protein vaccine that protects against strangles caused by Streptococcus equi. Vaccine 2018;36:1484–90.

65. Robinson C, Waller AS, Frykberg L, et al. Intramuscular vaccination with Strangvac is safe and induces protection against equine strangles caused by Streptococcus equi. Vaccine 2020;38(31):4861–8.

66. Ling AS, Upjohn MM, Webb K, et al. Seroprevalence of Streptococcus equi in working horses in Lesotho. Vet Rec 2011;169:72.

67. Tirosh-Levy S, Blum SE, Steward KF, et al. Streptococcus equi subspecies equi in horses in Israel: seroprevalence and strain types. Vet Rec Open 2016;3:e000187.

68. Libardoni F, Machado G, Gressler LT, et al. Prevalence of Streptococcus equi subsp. equi in horses and associated risk factors in the State of Rio Grande do Sul, Brazil. Res Vet Sci 2016;104:53–7.

69. McGlennon A, Waller A, Verheyen K, et al. Surveillance of strangles in UK horses between 2015 and 2019 based on laboratory detection of Streptococcus equi. Vet Rec 2021;189:e948.

70. Jorm LR. Laboratory studies on the survival of Streptococcus equi subspecies equi on surfaces. In: Plowright W, Rossdale PD, Wade JF, editors. Proceedings of equine infectious diseases VI. Newmarket, UK: R & W Publications Ltd; 1992. p. 39–43.

71. Weese JS, Jarlot C, Morley PS. Survival of Streptococcus equi on surfaces in an outdoor environment. Can Vet J 2009;50:968–70.

72. Durham AE, Hall YS, Kulp L, et al. A study of the environmental survival of Streptococcus equi subspecies equi. Equine Vet J 2018;50:861–4.

73. Pusterla N, Bowers J, Barnum S, et al. Molecular detection of Streptococcus equi subspecies equi in face flies (Musca autumnalis) collected during a strangles outbreak on a Thoroughbred farm. Med Vet Entomol 2020;34:120–2.

74. Svonni E, Andreasson M, Fernström LL, et al. Potential for residual contamination by Streptococcus equi subspp equi of endoscopes and twitches used in diagnosis of carriers of strangles. Equine Vet J 2020;52:884–90.

75. Torpiano P, Nestorova N, Vella C. Streptococcus equi subsp. equi meningitis, septicemia and subdural empyema in a child. IDCases 2020;21:e00808.

76. Willis AT, Barnum S, Pusterla N. Validation of a point-of-care polymerase chain reaction assay for detection of Streptococcus equi subspecies equi in rostral nasal swabs from horses with suspected strangles. Can Vet J 2021;62:51–4.

77. Boyle AG, Rankin SC, O'Shea K, et al. Detection of Streptococcus equi subsp. equi in guttural pouch lavage samples using a loop-mediated isothermal nucleic acid amplification microfluidic device. J Vet Intern Med 2021;35:1597–603.

78. Pusterla N, Barnum SM, Byrne BA. Investigation of a 24-Hour Culture Step to Determine the Viability of Streptococcus equi Subspecies equi Via Quantitative Polymerase Chain Reaction in Nasal Secretions From Horses With Suspected Strangles. J Equine Vet Sci 2021;97:103328.

79. Boyle AG, O'Shea K, Rankin SC. Propidium Monoazide - Quantitative Realtime Polymerase Chain Reaction for the Detection of Viable Streptococcus equi. In: ACVIM forum proceedings. 2018. Available at: https://www.vin.com/members/cms/project/defaultadv1.aspx?pId=20886&id=8524782. Accessed June 29, 2022.
80. Mitchell C, Steward KF, Charbonneau ARL, et al. Globetrotting strangles: the unbridled national and international transmission of Streptococcus equi between horses. Microb Genom 2021;7. https://doi.org/10.1099/mgen.0.000528. mgen000528.

Equine Granulocytic Anaplasmosis

Andrea Oliver, DVM[a], Francisco O. Conrado, DVM, MSc, DACVP[b],
Rose Nolen-Walston, DVM, ACVIM[a],*

KEYWORDS

- Horse • Granulocytic ehrlichiosis • Anaplasma phagocytophilum
- Tick-borne disease

KEY POINTS

- Equine granulocytic anaplasmosis is a common and clinically significant disease that is increasing due to changing climactic conditions.
- Typical clinical signs of fever and distal limb edema may be accompanied by less common clinical entities including neurologic and respiratory signs, among others.
- Multiple means of diagnosis are available including serologic testing, polymerase chain reaction, and direct organism visualization.
- Tetracycline antimicrobials are the most common treatment option alongside supportive care.
- No effective vaccine exists on the market. Tick prevention strategies are recommended for both human and equid health.

Abbreviations	
EGA	Equine granulocytic anaplasmosis
HGA	Human granulocytic anaplasmosis
CSF	cerebrospinal fluid
MSc	Master of Science
DACVIM	Diplomate of the American College of Veterinary Internal Medicine
DACVP	Diplomate of the American College of Veterinary Pathologists

INTRODUCTION

Equine granulocytic anaplasmosis (EGA) is an obligate intracellular, rickettsial disease of equids, humans, and other domestic species such as dogs, cats, sheep and cattle,

[a] Department of Clinical Studies, University of Pennsylvania, New Bolton Center, 382 West Street Road, Kennett Square, PA 19348, USA; [b] Department of Comparative Pathobiology, Tufts University, Cummings School of Veterinary Medicine, 200 Westboro Road, North Grafton, MA 01536, USA
* Corresponding author.
E-mail address: rnolenw@upenn.edu

Vet Clin Equine 39 (2023) 133–145
https://doi.org/10.1016/j.cveq.2022.11.011
0749-0739/23/© 2022 Elsevier Inc. All rights reserved.

as well as diverse wildlife species The disease is caused by the gram-negative, coc-cobacillary organism *Anaplasma phagocytophilum*. In 2001, multiple organisms infecting ruminants, horses, and humans, formerly known as *Ehrlichia phagocytophila*, *Ehrlichia equi*, and the then unnamed agent of human granulocytic ehrlichiosis under-went a taxonomic reclassification and were combined into a single species, *A phag-ocytophilum*. In fact, early work uniting these organisms was performed by veterinarians, who showed that a Thoroughbred filly inoculated with blood from a hu-man with granulocytic ehrlichiosis developed clinical signs consistent with equine granulocytic anaplasmosis and subsequently became resistant to challenge with *E equi*. Similar experiments were repeated with cattle, with the same result.[1,2]

The organism is transmitted by the ixodid tick, particularly during the late fall, winter, and spring. In endemic areas, EGA is a common and clinically significant disease of equids, which is encountered and treated in field and hospitalized settings. Changing climactic conditions have allowed for the persistence of arthropod vectors throughout the year and for geographic movement of the disease with its host to equids throughout the world.[3] The broad host tropism of the organism also raises concern for zoonotic potential, with domestic species serving as a reservoir, worsening spread of human granulocytic anaplasmosis (HGA). This review addresses current knowledge regarding the pathophysiology of EGA, recent developments in diagnosis and treat-ment, its less common clinical presentations, and an update on epidemiologic spread both geographically and across species.

PATHOGENESIS

Despite the prevalence of the disease, the entire pathogenesis of EGA has not been fully elucidated. The bacteria, *A phagocytophilum*, enters through the dermis via the bite of infected ticks. The usual vector is known to be the ixodid tick[4,5] among others,[6] specifically *Ixodes scapularis* and *Ixodes pacificus* in North America, as well as *Ixodes ricinus* in Europe. Small mammals, birds, and lizards may serve as reservoirs.[7] Although transovarial transmission seems to be possible in some ixodid species, rates are so low that the risk of infection by the larval tick stage is considered inconsequen-tial.[8] Therefore, the organism is maintained in reservoir hosts, including the white-footed mouse, *Peromyscus leucopus*, but also potentially the horse and other live-stock species.[9] During the larval or nymphal stage, the bacteria are acquired from a blood meal from an infected animal and then transmitted to a new host during the following nymphal or adult feeding. In mouse models, DNA of *A phagocytophilum* could be identified as early as 4 to 8 hours after attachment. Significant increases in both pathogen DNA detection and immunoglobulin response were noted during the 24-hour period, with most animals being infected after 36 hours of attachment.[10] Aside from transdermal transmission, only one case of transplacental transmission is reported in a foal, where a confirmed clinically affected mare produced a filly with compatible clinical signs and positive quantitative polymerase chain reaction (PCR) before ingestion of colostrum.[11]

Once through the dermis, the movement of the organism is still unclear. It is pre-sumed to travel via either the lymphatic system or blood and invade host neutrophils where replication occurs within vacuoles. The vacuole fails to fuse with lysosomes or neutrophil-specific granules, allowing for the replication of the organism and forma-tion of microcolonies termed "morulae,"[12] from the Latin word for "mulberry." The exact mechanism by which this is accomplished is incompletely understood; howev-er, recent evidence suggests that *A phagocytophilum* parasitizes portions of the endoplasmic reticulum to deliver packaged proteins to the vacuoles in which they reside. This pathogen-associated vacuole-endoplasmic reticulum interaction may help satisfy the nutritional requirements of the bacteria during leukocytic infection.[13] The organism lacks the genes for biosynthesis of factors that activate host leukocytes such as lipopolysaccharide and peptidoglycan. The lipopolysaccharide and peptidoglycan are acquired from acquisition of low-density lipoproteins produced by the cell to provide membrane stability.[14] A phagocytophilum also colonizes endothelial cells, providing a way to evade the immune system and spread to other leukocytes.[15]

The means by which host tissue destruction occurs still proves ambiguous, although may be related to neutrophilic oxidative and enzymatic processes that are typically initiated during phagocytosis. These processes are generally associated with tissue necrosis at the site of infection, which is not identified during transmission of A phagocytophilum. Across species, the heaviest burdens of infection are identified within the spleen, liver, and lungs, likely related to the early focal sequestration of infected cells. However, vasculitis seems to be a finding unique to equids.[12] Direct infection of hemoatopoeitic progenitor cells is unlikely to explain the associated pancytopenia noted in some human and ovid patients and thrombocytopenia recognized in horses, as the organism has not been commonly identified within the bone marrow. Peripheral sequestration, consumption, or destruction of blood elements is more likely.[12]

Infection with A phagocytophilum confers immunosuppressive effects to the host. Mammalian hosts show increased susceptibility to opportunistic infections during co-infection with A phagocytophilum, although this phenomenon is more commonly recognized in sheep than in horses[16]; this could be in part due to infection of the endothelium and subsequent alterations in its role in the inflammatory process. Alterations to both neutrophilic and lymphocytic function have also been suggested.[17]

In horses, clinical recovery ranges from a few days to several months. A chronic form has been suggested to exist in cases of prolonged recovery. The concept that this could be related to the immunosuppressive effects of the disease has been suggested, although not verified.[18]

EPIDEMIOLOGY

Prevalence of anaplasmosis seems to be spreading geographically in accordance with increasing climactic temperatures and prolongation of the vector season. There is significant variation in the epidemiology of this disease in North America and Europe.[19] HGA is common in humans in the United States, with 5000 to 6000 cases reported to the Centers of Disease Control and Prevention annually, yet it is apparently rare in Europe.[20] Conversely, tick-borne fever of sheep and cattle is common in Europe but not reported in North America, whereas granulocytic anaplasmosis of dogs, horses, and cats occurs on both continents. **Table 1** provides an updated summary of recent seroprevalence reports for A phagocytophilum in horses.

Clinical Signs

In equids, clinical signs of the acute syndrome include fever (generally 102–104°F)[45] along with concurrent depression, tachycardia occasionally alongside low-grade systolic murmurs, icterus, and anorexia.[46,47] Later in the course of disease, petechiation and distal limb edema may appear, alongside gait stiffness, myalgia, and sometimes overt lameness or unwillingness to move forward.[48]

Neurologic forms of the disease have also been reported, manifesting as mild hind limb ataxia[47,48] or more rarely as severe ataxia, which may persist further than 3 weeks

Table 1
Recent seroprevalence and antigen detection of *Anaplasma phagocytophilum* in horses globally

Country	Prevalence	Method of Identification	Comments	Reference
North America				
East Texas	65.7%, 28.6%	IFA, *msp2* qPCR	Healthy horses	Russell et al,[21] 2021
West Texas	66%, 0%	IFA, *msp2* qPCR	Healthy horses	Russell et al,[21] 2021
Central New York	100%, 8.2%	IFA, *msp2* qPCR	Healthy horses	Russell et al,[21] 2021
New Jersey	100%, 0%	IFA, *msp2* qPCR	Healthy horses	Russell et al,[21] 2021
Juarez, Mexico	0.8%	PCR	In horses with ticks removed	Medrano-Bugarini et al,[22] 2019
Canada	0.53%, 28.7%	ELISA SNAP 4Dx, IFA	Convenience serum submissions	Schvartz et al,[23] 2015
South America				
Brazil (Rio de Janeiro)	1.0%, 17.3%	*msp2* PCR, IFA	Healthy horses with and without ticks present	dos Santos et al,[24] 2019
Chile	7.9%, 13.6%	IFA, *msp2* rtPCR	Thoroughbred Racehorses	Hurtado et al,[25] 2020
Europe				
Ukraine	0.0%	Nested PCR	Healthy horses	Slivinska et al,[26] 2016
Ukraine	10%, 0%	PCR, Morulae identification	Horses with thrombocytopenia or compatible clinical signs	Dziegiel et al,[27] 2013
Poland	2.63%	Nested PCR	Polish primitive horses	Slivinska et al,[26] 2016
Poland	16.6%, 8.3%	PCR, Morulae identification	Horses with thrombocytopenia or compatible clinical signs	Dziegiel et al,[27] 2013
Romania	10.3%	ELISA Snap 4Dx	Healthy horses	Bogdan et al,[28] 2021
Turkey	8.57%	IFAT	Healthy race mares	Günaydin et al,[29] 2018
Italy (Northern)	23.4%	IFAT	Healthy horses	Villa et al,[30] 2022
Italy (Sicily)	9.0%, 4.7%	IFAT, PCR	Healthy horses	Giudice et al,[31] 2012
Italy	12.5%, 3.1%	PCR, Morulae identification	Horses with thrombocytopenia or compatible clinical signs	Dziegiel et al,[27] 2013

Location	Prevalence	Method	Horse type	Reference
Italy (Central)	17.03%, 8.14%	IFAT, nested PCR	Combined symptomatic and asymptomatic horses	Passamonti et al,[32] 2010
Spain	18.9%, 7.5%	PCR, Morulae identification	Horses with thrombocytopenia or compatible clinical signs	Dziegiel et al,[27] 2013
Germany	16.7%, 16.7%	PCR, Morulae identification	Horses with thrombocytopenia or compatible clinical signs	Dziegiel et al,[27] 2013
Germany	1.67%	PCR	Fever of unknown origin	von Loewenich et al,[33] 2003, Walls et al,[34] 1997
Netherlands	9.8%, 8.2	PCR, Morulae identification	Fever of unknown origin	Butler et al,[35] 2008
Netherlands	34%, 29.7%	IFAT, ELISA SNAP 4Dx	Horses with tick exposure	(Butler et al, 2016)
Bulgaria	20%	ELISA Snap 4Dx	Draft horses	Tsachev et al,[36] 2018
Denmark	22.3%	ELISA Snap 4Dx	Healthy horses	Hansen et al,[37] 2010
Sweden (southern)	32%	rtPCR	Horses with compatible clinical signs	Janzén et al,[38] 2019
Czech Republic	0.14%	IFA or PCR	Hospitalized horses	Jahn et al,[39] 2010
France	13.5%	ELISA SNAP 4Dx	Healthy horses	Maurizi et al,[40] 2009
Asia				
Iraq	28.9%	Morulae identification	Horses with compatible clinical signs	Albadrani & Al-Iraqi,[41] 2019
Pakistan	10.67%	PCR	Compatible clinical signs	Saleem et al,[42] 2018
Africa				
Tunisia	16.3%	IFAT	Healthy horses	ben Said et al,[43] 2014
Tunisia	67%, 13%	IFA, nPCR	Horses with and without ticks	Mghirbi et al,[44] 2012
Subsaharan Africa	0%	ELISA SNAP 4Dx	Healthy horses	Maurizi et al,[40] 2009

after initial infection.[49] In one case, ataxia was so severe as to progress to recumbency. In this case, cytologic evaluation of cerebrospinal fluid (CSF) was unremarkable.[50] One case report exists of a horse with areas of necrosis of the brain consistent with microinfarction and necrosis presumed to be associated with an infection with *A phagocytophilum* diagnosed based on PCR of both the blood and CSF. Diagnosis of microinfarction in this patient was initially suspected based on computed tomographic imaging of the brain.[51]

Other infrequently reported signs include upper respiratory disease with dysphagia described in 2 horses, one of which was diagnosed with laryngeal hemiplegia and one with diffuse pharyngeal edema. Speculated causation includes vasculitis and potentially associated peripheral neuritis, although this could not be confirmed.[52] In both cases, dysphagia resolved with treatment with tetracycline antibiotics. One case report also exists of 2 equids that presented with bicavitary effusion and hypoproteinemia, along with other signs compatible with anaplasmosis. The fluid was consistent with a serosanguinous effusion in one case and low-protein transudate in the other. *A phagocytophilum* was identified via PCR of both blood and effusion. In both cases, effusion and hypoproteinemia, along with other clinical signs of anaplasmosis, resolved with treatment with tetracycline antimicrobials.[53] Rhabdomyolysis has also been reported as an uncommon presentation of EGA. One horse was found with evidence of rhabdomyolysis that was positive for anaplasmosis on PCR of serum and muscle tissue. Muscle incisional biopsy showed histopathologic evidence that suggest oxidative stress and was not consistent with other common causes of rhabdomyolysis in quarter horses. This horse's clinical signs resolved after treatment with tetracycline antimicrobials.[54] In one experimentally infected case, the horse died, likely secondary to disseminated intravascular coagulopathy and circulatory collapse.[55] To date, fatal infections have not been reported within the naturally infected population.

The most commonly reported alteration of the hemogram noted with naturally occurring EGA is mild to moderate (but not severe) thrombocytopenia. However, in experimentally infected animals, transient pancytopenia was noted in the acute, febrile phase of the disease, with thrombocytopenia persisting longer. In general, lymphopenia and thrombocytopenia are most commonly reported.[48] Anecdotally, cytologic evidence of antigenic stimulation and the presence of reactive-appearing lymphocytes is frequently noted. Anemia is commonly identified in clinical cases. Bone marrow hypoplasia has been suggested to be the cause of these anemias.[45] On serum or plasma biochemistry, hyperbilirubinemia, hyponatremia, and hyperfibrinogenemia are common concurrent findings.[47]

Diagnosis

Visual identification of morulae within neutrophils can often be used as a simple, inexpensive diagnostic aid (**Fig. 1**). Morulae seem as small, intracytoplasmic clusters of blue-grey organisms within neutrophils on Wright-Giemsa–stained (or similar) blood smears, found especially within the feathered edge or in buffy coat preparations (**Fig. 2**). They can be identified as early as 2 to 4 days after onset of clinical disease. Identification of the characteristic morulae is specific for infection with *A phagocytophilum* in horses but is limited in sensitivity by the short window of appearance during clinical progress.[48] Anecdotally, buffy coat is likely to be more sensitive for identification of morulae than a direct blood smear based on the concentration of white blood cells. Absence of morulae should not be used to exclude anaplasmosis as a differential diagnosis, particularly early in the course of disease.

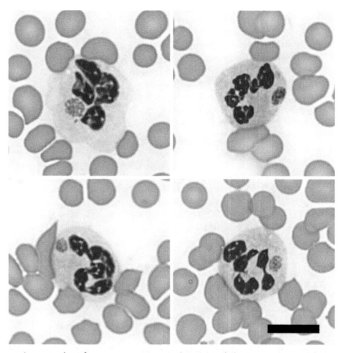

Fig. 1. Photomicrographs of mature, segmented neutrophils containing *A phagocytophilum* morulae on the blood smear from a 7-year-old Shetland Pony mare presented for evaluation of suspected strangles. Note the dotted appearance of the morulae, indicating the presence of several organisms (a vacuole-contained microcolony). Wright-Giemsa, bar = 10 μm.

Immunofluorescence assay (IFA) is commonly used to determine circulating antibodies to *A phagocytophilum* for the study of disease prevalence. Difficulty arises, however, when attempting to interpret seropositivity in the case of clinical cases. In one survey of an endemic area, 50% of healthy horses were identified as having titers to the organism in the absence of clinical disease.[56] Experimentally infected horses seroconverted by 12 to 16 days after inoculation, 2 days after the appearance of morulae on microscopic evaluation, and 8 days after the first positive PCR test result. In some cases, seroconversion occurred after the resolution of the horse's fever.[48] Based on this, a single titer is unlikely to provide clinical utility for the diagnosis of EGA in the face of disease, although it may provide evidence of past exposure. If paired serology is used, the first titer should be drawn early after clinical signs appear in order to document seroconversion after approximately 6 to 8 days. Smaller infective doses are suspected to induce a slower increase in antibody titers, so an additional titer could be drawn later in the course of disease, if the patient fails to seroconvert within the 6- to 8-day period. One earlier report after natural infection identified seroconversion as late as 19 to 81 days after infection.[57] Based on this time frame, failure to identify seroconversion should not rule out anaplasmosis.

A commercial enzyme-linked immunosorbent assay (ELISA) product for identification of antibodies to *A phagocytophilum* is available. Relative to IFA, although it is developed and marketed as a point-of-care test for canine samples, the SNAP 4Dx ELISA (IDEXX Laboratories) was 100% sensitive and specific for antibodies to *A phagocytophilum* in horses and could thus be considered a useful alternative to IFA.[37] As

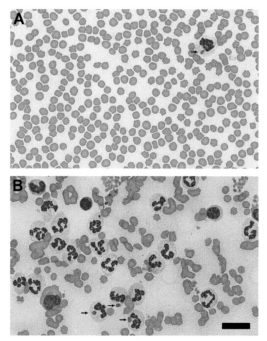

Fig. 2. Photomicrographs of the blood smear (*A*) and buffy coat preparation (*B*) from a 14-year-old Warmblood gelding presented for evaluation of acute colic. (*A*) An *A phagocytophilum* morula is seen within a neutrophil on the peripheral blood smear (*arrow*). A single neutrophil is seen within this high-magnification field. (*B*) Numerous leukocytes are seen in this concentrated preparation, including several containing *A phagocytophilum* morulae (*arrows*). Wright-Giemsa, bar = 20 μm.

with IFA, however, antibody detection may persist far beyond the period of clinical disease. One report suggests persistence of positive results via this modality as far as 9 months.[58]

PCR is positive as early as 3 days after inoculation with larger infective doses but may be as late as 5 to 6 days in animals with a smaller infective dose. In general, this is typically 2 to 3 days before the appearance of clinical signs.[48] Positive PCR results can persist as late as 129 days after infection, and horses may be intermittently positive consistent with stress induction. Based on these observations, the presence of persistent infection has been suggested, although no clinical signs associated with this positivity have been reported.[59]

Treatment

Tetracyclines are the most commonly used class of antimicrobials in treatment of anaplasmosis in horses. In-vitro studies show uniform susceptibility of *A phagocytophilum* to doxycycline.[60] Oxytetracycline at 3 to 24 mg/kg IVq12 to 24 hours,[11,33,49,52] doxycycline at 10 mg/kg PO q12 hours,[46] or minocycline at 4 mg/kg PO q12 hours[52] have been used with clinical success. However, self-limiting and subclinical disease may also exist, which could falsely increase perceived treatment success. Rifampin also shows efficacy against Anaplasma in vitro[60] and has been used with success in several human cases of HGA[61] and could be considered as an alternative in equine patients where concurrent renal disease presents concerns for tetracycline administration.

Alongside antimicrobials, supportive care includes using nonsteroidal antiinflammatory drugs, acetaminophen, or opioids to manage pain associated with edema and myalgia. Steroids have been occasionally used in severe cases. In experimentally infected animals, dexamethasone (40 mg/horse) was shown to reduce proinflammatory cytokines associated with infection with concurrent reductions in distal limb edema, icterus, anorexia, reluctance to move in later disease, and fever on day 7. Notably, peripheral blood load based on quantitative PCR of *A phagocytophilum* was shown to increase in the face of dexamethasone treatment despite clinical improvement, supporting the importance of inflammatory factor release in disease pathogenesis.[62]

Prevention

No vaccine exists on the market for anaplasmosis, currently. Thus, prevention mainly consists of careful environmental maintenance to reduce exposure to ticks. Horses in endemic areas should have limited exposure to forested areas, overgrown grasses, and shrubberies where ticks are abundant. Properties should also be cleared of debris and stone-wall structures, which are associated with increased tick populations.[63] Measures should also be taken to reduce the number of small rodents in the area by keeping grain products carefully stowed and storage areas regularly cleaned.

As anaplasmosis infectivity is known to increase with the length of attachment time,[10] regular tick checks should be conducted to remove new ticks as rapidly as possible. The ear canals and tail should be carefully investigated. Permethrin products have been shown to hinder normal tick movement and so can also be considered for regular usage in equine patients during the vector season.[64] Anecdotally, fipronil spray of the distal limbs and tail may be an efficacious alternative.

Zoonotic Potential

Although EGA is not directly transmissible from equids to humans, equine patients may serve as a reservoir for disease persistence through seasons of decreased tick activity. Equids may harbor strains of the same clonal complex identified in human cases of HGA.[65] Typical clinical signs in humans include flulike symptoms 2 weeks after inoculation, with severity worsening in the immunosuppressed population. Thus, prompt disease identification and treatment in the equine patient is necessary to reduce spread and infective potential of ticks in the environment. With this in mind, ticks that are removed from horses should be carefully destroyed to avoid possibility of reattachment onto human hosts.

SUMMARY

Equine granulocytic anaplasmosis is a clinically significant disease of horses, with the same cause causing disease in many other domesticated animals, and humans, with a broader prevalence than once thought. Early disease identification using clinical signs and appropriate confirmatory testing is important for the initiation of rapid treatment and recovery. The most common clinical signs include fever, edema, petechia, icterus, depression, and anorexia; however, subclinical cases are reported, and many infections are self-limiting. Anaplasmosis should be considered in cases of suspected vasculitis or neurologic disease, which cannot be attributed to other agents, particularly as most cases resolve well with appropriate antimicrobial intervention. As the vector season of tick populations increases and transport of animals is more easily facilitated, consideration for the human health implications of anaplasmosis should be considered in managing equine populations.

CLINICAL CARE POINTS

- Many cases of equine granulocytic anaplasmosis are subclinical or self-limiting.
- Most cases respond rapidly and completely to tetracycline antimicrobials and supportive care.
- Anaplasmosis should be considered in cases of neurologic disease, vasculitis, dysphagia, rhabdomyolysis, or bicavitary effusion associated with hypoproteinemia, which cannot be otherwise explained.
- Seroprevalence varies significantly by geographic region, and seropositivity is prolonged after exposure. Diagnosis is best made by paired serology, PCR, or visualization of the organism on blood smear.

DISCLOSURE

The authors have nothing to disclose.

REFERENCES

1. Barlough JE, Madigan JE, DeRock E, et al. Protection against Ehrlichia equi is conferred by prior infection with the human granulocytotropic Ehrlichia (HGE agent). J Clin Microbiol 1995;33(12):3333–4.
2. Pusterla N, Anderson RJ, House JK, et al. Susceptibility of cattle to infection with Ehrlichia equi and the agent of human granulocytic ehrlichiosis. J Am Vet Med Assoc 2001;218(7):1160–2.
3. Laus F, Veronesi F, Passamonti F, et al. Prevalence of tick borne pathogens in horses from Italy. J Vet Med Sci 2013;75(6):715–20.
4. Pusterla N, Chae JS, Kimsey RB, et al. Transmission of Anaplasma phagocytophila (Human Granulocytic Ehrlichiosis Agent) in Horses Using Experimentally Infected Ticks (Ixodes scapularis). J Vet Med Ser B 2002;49(10):484–8.
5. Reubel GH, Kimsey RB, Barlough JE, et al. Experimental transmission of Ehrlichia equi to horses through naturally infected ticks (Ixodes pacificus) from Northern California. J Clin Microbiol 1998;36(7):2131–4.
6. Price KJ, Ayres BN, Maes SE, et al. First detection of human pathogenic variant of Anaplasma phagocytophilum in field-collected Haemaphysalis longicornis, Pennsylvania, USA. Zoonoses and Public Health 2022;69(2):143–8.
7. Nieto NC, Madigan JE, Foley JE. The dusky-footed woodrat (Neotoma fuscipes) is susceptible to infection by Anaplasma phagocytophilum originating from woodrats, horses, and dogs. J Wildl Dis 2010;46(3):810–7.
8. Hauck D, Jordan D, Springer A, et al. Transovarial transmission of Borrelia spp., Rickettsia spp. And Anaplasma phagocytophilum in Ixodes ricinus under field conditions extrapolated from DNA detection in questing larvae. Parasites and Vectors 2020;13(1):1–11.
9. Ravyn MD, Kodner CB, Carter SE, et al. Isolation of the etiologic agent of human granulocytic ehrlichiosis from the white-footed mouse (Peromyscus leucopus). J Clin Microbiol 2001;39(1):335–8.
10. Levin ML, Troughton DR, Loftis AD. Duration of tick attachment necessary for transmission of Anaplasma phagocytophilum by Ixodes scapularis (Acari: Ixodidae) nymphs. Ticks Tick-Borne Dis 2021;12(6):101819.

11. Dixon CE, Bedenice D. Transplacental infection of a foal with Anaplasma phago-cytophilum. Equine Vet Education 2021;33(3):e62–6.
12. Rikihisa Y. Mechanisms of obligatory intracellular infection with Anaplasma phag-ocytophilum. Clin Microbiol Rev 2011;24(3):469–89.
13. Truchan HK, Cockburn CL, Hebert KS, et al. The Pathogen-Occupied Vacuoles of Anaplasma phagocytophilum and Anaplasma marginale Interact with the Endo-plasmic Reticulum. Front Cell Infect Microbiol 2016;6(MAR):22.
14. Lin M, Rikihisa Y. Ehrlichia chaffeensis and Anaplasma phagocytophilum lack genes for lipid A biosynthesis and incorporate cholesterol for their survival. Infect Immun 2003;71(9):5324–31.
15. Herron MJ, Ericson ME, Kurtti TJ, et al. The Interactions of Anaplasma phagocy-tophilum, Endothelial Cells, and Human Neutrophils. Ann N Y Acad Sci 2005; 1063(1):374–82.
16. Granquist EG, Stuen S, Lundgren AM, et al. Outer membrane protein sequence variation in lambs experimentally infected with Anaplasma phagocytophilum. Infect Immun 2008;76(1):120–6.
17. Woldehiwet Z. Immune evasion and immunosuppression by Anaplasma phago-cytophilum, the causative agent of tick-borne fever of ruminants and human gran-ulocytic anaplasmosis. Vet J 2008;175(1):37–44.
18. Artursson K, Gunnarsson A, Wikström UB, et al. A serological and clinical follow-up in horses with confirmed equine granulocytic ehrlichiosis. Equine Vet J 1999; 31(6):473–7.
19. Scharf W, Schauer S, Freyburger F, et al. Distinct Host Species Correlate with Anaplasma phagocytophilum ankA Gene Clusters. J Clin Microbiol 2011; 49(3):790.
20. Epidemiology and Statistics | Anaplasmosis. CDC 2021. Available at: https://www.cdc.gov/anaplasmosis/stats/index.html.
21. Russell A, Shost N, Burch M, et al. Serological and Molecular Detection of Ana-plasma spp. in Blood From Healthy Horses: A Preliminary Study of Horses in East Texas. J Equine Vet Sci 2021;106. https://doi.org/10.1016/J.JEVS.2021.103757.
22. Medrano-Bugarini RA, Figueroa-Millán JV, Rivera-Chavira BE, et al. Detection of Theileria equi, Babesia caballi, and Anaplasma phagocytophilum DNA in Soft Ticks and Horses at Ciudad Juarez, Mexico 2019;44(3):647–58.
23. Schvartz G, Epp T, Burgess HJ, et al. Seroprevalence of equine granulocytic anaplasmosis and lyme borreliosis in Canada as determined by a point-of-care enzyme-linked immunosorbent assay (ELISA). Can Vet J 2015;56(6):575.
24. dos Santos TM, Roier ECR, Pires MS, et al. Molecular evidence of Anaplasma phagocytophilum and Theileria equi coinfection in horses from Rio de Janeiro, Brazil. Vet Anim Sci 2019;7:100055.
25. Hurtado C, Torres R, Pérez-Macchi S, et al. Serological and molecular detection of Anaplasma phagocytophilum in Thoroughbred horses from Chilean race-courses. Ticks Tick-Borne Dis 2020;11(4). https://doi.org/10.1016/J.TTBDIS.2020.101441.
26. Slivinska K, Víchová B, Werszko J, et al. Molecular surveillance of Theileria equi and Anaplasma phagocytophilum infections in horses from Ukraine, Poland and Slovakia. Vet Parasitol 2016;215:35–7.
27. Dziegiel B, Adaszek L, Winiarczyk M, et al. Comparative analysis of 16S RNA nucleotide sequences of Anaplasma phagocytophilum detected in the blood of horses from various parts of Europe. J Med Microbiol 2013;62(Pt 12):1891–6.
28. Bogdan AM, Ionita M, Mitrea IL. Serological Evidence of Natural Exposure to Tick-Borne Pathogens in Horses, Romania. Microorganisms 2021;9(2):373.

29. Günaydin E, Pekkaya S, Kuzugüden F, et al. The first detection of anti-anaplasma phagocytophilum antibodies in horses in Turkey. Kafkas Universitesi Veteriner Fakultesi Dergisi 2018;24(6):867–71.

30. Villa L, Gazzonis AL, Allievi C, et al. Seroprevalence of Tick-Borne Infections in Horses from Northern Italy. Animals (Basel) 2022;12(8):999.

31. Giudice E, Giannetto C, Furco V, et al. Anaplasma phagocytophilum seroprevalence in equids: a survey in Sicily (Italy). Parasitol Res 2012;111(2):951–5.

32. Passamonti F, Veronesi F, Cappelli K, et al. Anaplasma phagocytophilum in horses and ticks: a preliminary survey of Central Italy. Comp Immunol Microbiol Infect Dis 2010;33(1):73–83.

33. von Loewenich FD, Stumpf G, Baumgarten BU, et al. A case of equine granulocytic ehrlichiosis provides molecular evidence for the presence of pathogenic anaplasma phagocytophilum (HGE agent) in Germany. Eur J Clin Microbiol Infect Dis 2003;22(5):303–5.

34. Walls JJ, Greig B, Neitzel DF, et al. Natural infection of small mammal species in Minnesota with the agent of human granulocytic ehrlichiosis. J Clin Microbiol 1997;35(4):853–5.

35. Butler CM, Nijhof AM, Jongejan F, et al. Anaplasma phagocytophilum infection in horses in the Netherlands. Vet Rec 2008;162(7):216–8.

36. Tsachev I, Pantchev N, Marutsov P, et al. Serological Evidence of Borrelia burgdorferi, Anaplasma phagocytophilum and Ehrlichia Spp. Infections in Horses from Southeastern Bulgaria. Vector Borne Zoonotic Dis (Larchmont, N.Y.) 2018; 18(11):588–94.

37. Hansen MGB, Christoffersen M, Thuesen LR, et al. Seroprevalence of Borrelia burgdorferi sensu lato and Anaplasma phagocytophilum in Danish horses. Acta Vet Scand 2010;52(1). https://doi.org/10.1186/1751-0147-52-3.

38. Janzén T, Petersson M, Hammer M, et al. Equine Granulocytic Anaplasmosis in Southern Sweden: Associations with coniferous forest, water bodies and landscape heterogeneity. Agric Ecosyst Environ 2019;285:106626.

39. Jahn P, Zeman P, Bezdekova B, et al. Equine granulocytic anaplasmosis in the Czech Republic. Vet Rec 2010;166(21):646–9.

40. Maurizi L, Marié JL, Courtin C, et al. Seroprevalence survey of equine anaplasmosis in France and in sub-Saharan Africa. Clin Microbiol Infect 2009; 15(SUPPL. 2):68–9.

41. Albadrani BA, Al-Iraqi OM. First detection of equine anaplasmosis and hemoplasmosis of horses in Mosul City, Iraq. Adv Anim Vet Sci 2019;7(2):106–11.

42. Saleem S, Ijaz M, Farooqi SH, et al. First molecular evidence of equine granulocytic anaplasmosis in Pakistan. Acta Trop 2018;180:18–25.

43. ben Said M, Belkahia H, Mejed Héni M, et al. Seroprevalence of Anaplasma phagocytophilum in well-maintained horses from northern Tunisia. Trop Biomed 2014;31(3):432–40.

44. Mghirbi Y, Yach H, Ghorbel A, et al. Anaplasma phagocytophilum in horses and ticks in Tunisia. Parasites and Vectors 2012;5(1):1–7.

45. Madigan JE, Gribble D. Equine ehrlichiosis in northern California: 49 cases (1968-1981). J Am Vet Med Assoc 1987;190(4):445–8. Available at: https:// pubmed.ncbi.nlm.nih.gov/3558086/.

46. Lewis SR, Zimmerman K, Dascanio JJ, et al. Equine Granulocytic Anaplasmosis: A Case Report and Review. J Equine Vet Sci 2009;29(3):160–6.

47. Siska WD, Tuttle RE, Messick JB, et al. Clinicopathologic Characterization of Six Cases of Equine Granulocytic Anaplasmosis In a Nonendemic Area (2008-2011). J Equine Vet Sci 2013;33(8):653–7.

48. Franzén P, Aspan A, Egenvall A, et al. Acute Clinical, Hematologic, Serologic, and Polymerase Chain Reaction Findings in Horses Experimentally Infected with a European Strain of Anaplasma phagocytophilum. J Vet Intern Med 2005;19(2):232–9.
49. Gussmann K, Czech C, Hermann M, et al. Anaplasma phagocytophilum infection in a horse from Switzerland with severe neurological symptoms. Schweizer Archiv Fur Tierheilkunde 2014;156(7):345–8.
50. Nolen-Walston RD, D'oench SM, Hanelt LM, et al. Acute recumbency associated with Anaplasma phagocytophilum infection in a horse. J Am Vet Med Assoc 2004; 224(12):1964–6.
51. Nowicka B, Polkowska I, Adaszek L, et al. Horse anaplasmosis as a cause of CNS infections and the use of computed tomography as a diagnostic imaging tool to present of its cerebral form: literature review supplemented with a clinical case. Med Weter 2022;78(5):239–43.
52. Deane EL, Fielding CL, Rhodes DM, et al. Upper respiratory signs associated with Anaplasma phagocytophilum infection in two horses. Equine Vet Education 2021;33(3):e58–61.
53. Restifo MM, Bedenice D, Thane KE, et al. Cavitary Effusion Associated with Anaplasma phagocytophilum Infection in 2 Equids. J Vet Intern Med 2015;29(2):732.
54. Hilton H, Madigan IE, Aleman M. Rhabdomyolysis Associated with Anaplasma phagocytophilum Infection in a Horse. J Vet Intern Med 2008;22(4):1061–4.
55. Franzén P, Berg AL, Aspan A, et al. Death of a horse infected experimentally with Anaplasma phagocytophilum. Vet Rec 2007;160(4):122–5.
56. Madigan JE, Hietala S, Chalmers S, et al. Seroepidemiologic survey of antibodies to Ehrlichia equi in horses of northern California. J Am Vet Med Assoc 1990; 196(12):1962–4. Available at: https://europepmc.org/article/med/2195000.
57. van Andel AE, Magnarelli LA, Heimer R, et al. Development and duration of antibody response against Ehrlichia equi in horses. J Am Vet Med Assoc 1998; 212(12):1910–4. Available at: https://europepmc.org/article/med/9638192.
58. Johnson AL, Divers TJ, Chang YF. Validation of an in-clinic enzyme-linked immunosorbent assay kit for diagnosis of Borrelia burgdorferi infection in horses. J Vet Diagn Invest 2008;20(3):321–4.
59. Franzén P, Aspan A, Egenvall A, et al. Molecular evidence for persistence of Anaplasma phagocytophilum in the absence of clinical abnormalities in horses after recovery from acute experimental infection. J Vet Intern Med 2009;23(3):636–42.
60. Maurin M, Bakken JS, Dumler JS. Antibiotic Susceptibilities of Anaplasma (Ehrlichia) phagocytophilum Strains from Various Geographic Areas in the United States. Antimicrob Agents Chemother 2003;47(1):413.
61. Buitrago MI, Ijdo JW, Rinaudo P, et al. Human granulocytic ehrlichiosis during pregnancy treated successfully with rifampin. Clin Infect Dis 1998;27(1):213–5.
62. Davies RS, Madigan JE, Hodzic E, et al. Dexamethasone-Induced Cytokine Changes Associated with Diminished Disease Severity in Horses Infected with Anaplasma phagocytophilum. Clin Vaccin Immunol : CVI 2011;18(11):1962.
63. Fischhoff IR, Keesing F, Pendleton J, et al. Assessing Effectiveness of Recommended Residential Yard Management Measures Against Ticks. J Med Entomol 2019;56(5):1420.
64. Prose R, Breuner NE, Johnson TL, et al. Contact Irritancy and Toxicity of Permethrin-Treated Clothing for Ixodes scapularis, Amblyomma americanum, and Dermacentor variabilis Ticks (Acari: Ixodidae). J Med Entomol 2018;55(5): 1217–24.
65. Stuen S, Granquist E, Silaghi C. Anaplasma phagocytophilum - pathogen with a zoonotic potential. Parasites & Vectors 2014;7(Suppl 1):O24.

Vesicular Stomatitis Virus

Angela M. Pelzel-McCluskey, DVM, MS

KEYWORDS

- Vesicular stomatitis • Livestock disease • Equine • Vector-borne disease outbreak

KEY POINTS

- Vesicular stomatitis (VS) is a disease reportable to state and federal animal health officials in the United States. Veterinarians suspecting VS in a clinical animal should contact either the State Veterinarian or the federal Area Veterinarian in Charge (AVIC) for the state in which the animal is located.
- Diagnostic confirmation of vesicular stomatitis virus (VSV) infection at an approved laboratory is required for the first equine case in a county and in all suspected cases in ruminants and swine.
- Isolation of animals with lesions and implementation of aggressive vector control measures are imperative to reduce the spread of VSV during an outbreak.
- VSV is a zoonotic pathogen that can be transmitted to humans through direct contact with animals with lesions. Personal protective equipment and good biosecurity practices should be used by veterinarians and animal handlers when handling horses and other livestock with active VS lesions.

INTRODUCTION

Vesicular stomatitis (VS) is a viral, vector-borne disease of livestock caused by *Vesiculoviruses,* vesicular stomatitis New Jersey virus (VSNJV) or vesicular stomatitis Indiana virus (VSIV), referred to collectively as vesicular stomatitis viruses (VSV). The disease is confined to the Americas where it occurs annually in endemic cycles in Mexico, Central America, and northern regions of South America and only in sporadic epizootic outbreaks every 2 to 10 years in the United States.[1] Equids, such as horses, mules, and donkeys, are the most commonly affected species in US outbreaks, followed by cattle and camelids, such as llamas and alpacas[2]; however, the disease can also occur in other ruminants and swine. Clinical signs of the disease in affected species are produced by the development of vesicular (blister-like) lesions that occur on the muzzle, nostrils, lips, oral mucosa, tongue, teats, udder, sheath, ventral abdomen, ears, and/or coronary bands (**Fig. 1**).[3] Lesions in the mouth and on the tongue usually cause hypersalivation and anorexia, whereas coronary band lesions often produce lameness. The disease is self-limiting and the lesions in most affected

United States Department of Agriculture, Animal and Plant Health Inspection Service, Veterinary Services, 2150 Centre Avenue, Building B, Fort Collins, CO, 80526, USA
E-mail address: Angela.M.Pelzel-McCluskey@usda.gov

Vet Clin Equine 39 (2023) 147–155
https://doi.org/10.1016/j.cveq.2022.11.004   **vetequine.theclinics.com**
0749-0739/23/Published by Elsevier Inc.

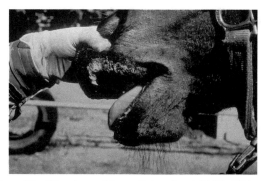

Fig. 1. Vesicular stomatitis. (*Courtesy* of Jason E. Lombard, DVM, MS.)

livestock heal within a couple of weeks without veterinary intervention; however, some older animals or those with underlying health conditions may require supportive care, especially in cases with severe oral lesions where the animals cease to eat or drink.[3] The disease is also zoonotic, transmitted to humans through direct contact with infectious lesions in livestock, and typically causes fever, headache, fatigue, and myalgia lasting 3 to 5 days.[3] The appearance of VSV-caused lesions in ruminants and swine is clinically indistinguishable from lesions of foot and mouth disease (FMD), one of the most economically devastating viral diseases of livestock[1]; therefore, immediate reporting to state and federal animal health officials of VSV-like lesions is required in the United States to first rule out FMD infection using appropriate diagnostic assays.

Transmission of VSV to horses and other livestock species occurs mainly through biting insects[4]; however, the spread can also occur through direct contact with virus-containing fluids from infectious lesions and saliva or through indirect contact with contaminated fomites, such as shared water, feed, feeders, lick tubs, tack, or veterinary supplies, like oral drenching equipment or dental floats.[5,6] Suspected vectors of VSV include black flies (Simuliidae), sand flies (Psychodidae), and *Culicoides* biting midges (Ceratopogonidae) as species from all three of these families have been found naturally infected with VSV in the wild.[7–9] However, other biting insects have been experimentally infected with VSV and may also be involved in transmission. Proximity of affected livestock premises to water has been indicated as a significant risk factor, which is likely reflective of nearness to prime habitat for competent vectors.[10] Black flies, hatching from moving waterways, and *Culicoides spp.*, hatching from muddy areas around standing water, move directly to nearby livestock to feed, thus initiating VSV transmission in the area if those vector populations are carrying the virus.

Genetic analyses of VSVs from US outbreaks have indicated that they arise from viruses circulating in Mexico.[11–13] Both VSV serotypes and multiple lineages are found circulating in southern and south-central Mexico annually.[1,13,14] It is hypothesized that specific climatic and environmental factors occur in certain years that favor expansion of VSV-carrying vectors northward from these endemic regions. In those years, VS cases are seen in states in northern Mexico just a few months before outbreaks being recognized in Texas, New Mexico, and/or Arizona in the United States. These years have been termed incursion years for US outbreaks, and the dominant climatological and ecological variables supporting this movement have been modeled and reported.[15] After an incursion year, the virus may overwinter and resurge to cause cases the following year, termed an expansion year, with slightly different climatological and ecological conditions identified as supporting this resurgence.[15] Northward expansion has been documented in horses as far north as Montana [https://www.aphis.usda. gov/vs/nahss/equine/vsv/vsvmaps/MT_2005_Cumulative_Final_121105.pdf]. If no VS outbreak is identified in the year following an incursion year, then it is hypothesized that the environmental variables supporting the vectors for an expansion year may not have been present and therefore, the continued transmission did not occur. Research is ongoing to further evaluate and understand how climate and ecology affect insect vector populations and the potential for VSV transmission in a given year.

VS outbreaks in the United States cause significant trade disruptions and economic impacts, mainly through cessation of international and interstate movement of live-stock, but also through reduced participation in or cancellation of equine and live-stock shows and events.[16] The seasonality of disease occurrence also has an impact. VS outbreaks occur during the height of vector activity, usually late spring through early fall, which is also the time of year where a high volume of equine shows/events and county fairs are scheduled to occur. In addition, the large numbers of cattle in the western United States that move through livestock markets and sales in the fall can be held up by VS outbreaks and associated quarantines. States without VS cases issue specific movement restrictions on susceptible livestock species from VS-affected states which may bar movement from affected counties altogether or require a certificate of veterinary inspection within just a few days of movement that includes statements by the veterinarian attesting to the examination of the animal and the absence of VS lesions. International export of livestock from VS-affected states is halted until at least 30 days after the last quarantine release in the state or longer depending on the requirements of the receiving country. International export of livestock from non-affected US states is usually able to proceed; however testing for VSV may be required by the receiving country which adds additional planning and expense to the exporters. Although the World Organization for Animal Health (WOAH) (formerly Office International des Epizooties [OIE]) removed VS from its list of interna-tionally reportable diseases in 2015, the United States remains bound by bilateral trade agreements with its trade partners to immediately report the occurrence of VS and provide information on response measures and updates on the outbreak.

History and Management of the Disease in the United States

Over the past 20 years, VS outbreaks in the United States have been geographically confined mainly to the southwestern and Rocky Mountain regions of the country, have primarily involved the VSNJV serotype of the virus, and large multi-year out-breaks have been temporally separated in 4- to 8-year increments with smaller, single incursion outbreak years occurring sporadically in between. A summary of outbreak years, affected states, virus serotype, and number of affected livestock premises dur-ing this time period is presented in **Table 1**. Historically, equine premises make up the majority of the affected premises identified during each outbreak year. Several factors may be involved in why equine premises are most impacted during an outbreak, such as vector preference for equids and/or common management practices on equine premises. For example, daily feeding and handling practices on equine premises make it more likely that clinically affected horses will be noticed by owners or barn managers, as opposed to grazing cattle operations where the animals may not be observed directly for days or weeks at a time, and even when observed, may not be noticed to have a clinical abnormality. In the Rocky Mountain region of the United States, many cattle herds are moved to high mountain pastures for the summer months and will not be physically observed until gathered again in the fall. Equine

Table 1
Summary of vesicular stomatitis outbreaks in the United States within the past 20 y including outbreak year, affected states, virus serotype, and number of affected livestock premises

Outbreak Year	Number of States Affected	States	VSV Serotype	Number of Affected Premises
2004	3	CO, NM, TX	VSNJV	294
2005	9	AZ, CO, ID, MT, NE, NM, TX, UT, WY	VSNJV	445
2006	1	WY	VSNJV	13
2009	2	NM, TX	VSNJV	5
2010	1	AZ	VSNJV	2
2012	2	CO, NM	VSNJV	36
2014	4	AZ, CO, NE, TX	VSNJV	435
2015	8	AZ, CO, NE, NM, SD, TX, UT, WY	VSNJV	823
2019	8	CO, KS, NE, NM, OK, TX, UT, WY	VSIV	1,144
2020	8	AR, AZ, KS, MO, NE, NM, OK, TX	VSIV, VSNJV (TX)	326

Abbreviations: AR, arkansas; AZ, arizona; CO, colorado; ID, idaho; KS, kansas; MO, missouri; MT, montana; NE, nebraska; NM, new mexico; OK, oklahoma; SD, south dakota; TX, texas; UT, utah; WY, wyoming.

owners are also more likely to seek veterinary care in response to noticing a clinical abnormality in their horse(s).

Ongoing surveillance for FMD and other foreign vesicular diseases of concern in the United States requires that United States Department of Agriculture (USDA)-accredited private veterinarians immediately report to state and federal animal health officials on suspected vesicular lesion occurrence in all livestock species, including equids. Follow-up on each report is conducted by a local state or federal veterinary medical officer specifically trained as a foreign animal disease diagnostician (FADD) who deploys to the affected livestock premises, examines the animals, collects the appropriate diagnostic samples, and places a quarantine on the premises. Diagnostic samples are shipped overnight to the USDA's National Veterinary Services Laboratories (NVSL) in either Ames, Iowa, or Plum Island, New York, depending on the species affected. Samples from equids with vesicular lesions, which cannot be infected with FMD, go to NVSL in Ames, Iowa, with diagnostic testing for VS as the primary rule out. Samples from ruminants and swine with lesions go to NVSL on Plum Island for primary rule out of FMD and foreign swine vesicular diseases, followed by secondary rule out of VS, and tertiary testing for domestic vesicular diseases, such as bluetongue, epizootic hemorrhagic disease, and bovine papular stomatitis in cattle and Senecavirus A in swine.

In all suspect cases, samples to be collected from animals with lesions include a serum sample and swabs of the lesions submitted in viral transport media. Diagnostic assays at NVSL used to confirm VSV infection are specific to each VSV serotype and include antibody detection methods on serum samples, such as competitive enzyme-linked immunosorbent assay (cELISA), complement fixation test (CFT), virus neutralization (VN), and virus detection methods on swab samples, such as real-time reverse transcription polymerase chain reaction (rRT-PCR) and virus isolation (VI). Although the cELISA is an early indicator of recent infection and will test positive a few days before the CFT in a naïve, recently exposed animal, the cELISA may subsequently remain positive for up to 10 to 12 years.[17] Given the number of previously exposed livestock residing in historically affected regions in the United States, the cELISA alone cannot be used to confirm recent infection unless occurring in an animal that was either not geographically present in a previous outbreak region or in an animal too young to have experienced the last US outbreak. The CFT, rRT-PCR, and/or VI are used as reliable indicators of recent infection for the purposes of VS case definition during an outbreak. All case definitions for VS require compatible clinical signs and have several options for diagnostic confirmation using these assays. An IgM capture ELISA has been developed recently at NVSL and may also be used as a reliable indicator of recent infection in future outbreaks. Although the VS index case for the nation, index cases for newly affected states, and VS cases in ruminants and swine require diagnostic confirmation at NVSL, since 2015 the USDA-approved National Animal Health Laboratory Network (NAHLN) laboratories located in historically VS-affected states have been activated during outbreaks to conduct VSV testing in clinically-affected equids. This action has successfully increased laboratory capacity and reduced result turnaround time during an outbreak response.

Once an index case of VS is diagnostically confirmed in the United States, a national situation report is issued first to state and federal animal health officials and bilateral trade partners for their awareness and then the report is publicly posted to the USDA-APHIS website.[2] At least once weekly situation reports are issued and posted throughout the outbreak thereafter until the incident is declared over, usually 30 days after the last quarantine release in the country. A joint state–federal response following standardized response protocols and using local personnel is organized in each affected state. A national-level situation unit leader is activated to provide support, maintain response continuity across states, gather data, and issue situation reports. State animal health officials provide electronic communication by mass email to private veterinarians licensed to practice in the state notifying them of the confirmation of a VS case, recommending increased surveillance and educational outreach to clients, reminding of reporting requirements, and providing instructions on response measures. Information is also posted to state animal health officials' websites, including specifics of any new interstate movement and entry requirements enacted as a response measure.

Livestock premises with laboratory diagnostic results meeting a VS confirmed case definition are categorized as confirmed positive premises. Once a county is confirmed as VSV-positive, new equine premises presenting with clinical signs of VSV in that county are not required to be tested for confirmation of the disease, but the premises are quarantined and classified as suspect premises. Premises are also classified as suspect if clinical animals on the premises fail to meet a confirmed case definition, but have diagnostic evidence of recent VSV infection. All confirmed positive and suspect VS premises are placed under state quarantine for a minimum of 14 days from the onset of lesions in the last affected animal on the premises. The quarantine applies to all VS-susceptible species on the premises and no movement of these species off-site is permitted without approval of the state veterinarian.

Isolation of animals with lesions from clinically healthy animals is instituted to reduce spread of the virus by direct contact, and aggressive vector control recommendations are provided to be instituted by the premises/animal owner to further reduce within-herd spread. Oversight for equine premises is conducted by private veterinarians communicating with state animal health officials in most states, whereas oversight of ruminant and swine premises is conducted directly by state or federal animal health officials. Private veterinarians or animal health officials overseeing each premises confirm the 14-day countdown after the onset of lesions in the last affected animal. State animal health officials issue a quarantine release once this time period has passed with no new cases presenting. Continuation of aggressive vector control on the premises is recommended throughout the remainder of the outbreak, as re-infection of previously affected animals and lesion development in new animals after quarantine release has occurred occasionally from continued presence of infected vectors in the general area when vector mitigations on the premises are inadequate.

DISCUSSION

Recent outbreaks of VS in the United States have provided evidence that climate change may be impacting the future size, scope, and geographic range of outbreaks. The 2019 and 2020 VS outbreaks shared some characteristic features of historic outbreaks in the United States, but also had several unexpected attributes potentially related to climatic factors. The 2019 VSIV outbreak resulted in identification of 1,144 VSV-affected premises in 111 counties in eight states. The factors involved that boosted this outbreak to become the largest in both size and geographic scope in the past 40 years of recorded history are still a relative mystery, although climatological and ecological conditions affecting vector abundance, dispersal, or habitat quality are suspected to be involved. Indeed, the previous round of outbreaks in 2014 to 2015 was also larger than normal by comparison to other years and may hold the key to identification of climate factors that may have been intensifying into 2019. Questions remain regarding what caused US outbreaks to be dominated exclusively by the VSNJV serotype since the last VSIV outbreak in 1997 to 1998 and, subsequently, what changed that allowed VSIV to appear and surge alone so successfully in 2019. Clinically, the VSNJV and VSIV presented across the outbreaks quite similarly with the full gamut of lesion types represented and neither virus serotype looking any more or less virulent in the animals than the other.

Phylogenetic analysis supports the occurrence of an overwintering event of VSIV between the 2019 and 2020 outbreaks.[18] Although overwintering of the virus was an expected event based on historic occurrences of the same pattern, there were several completely unexpected outcomes that followed. Based on study of the 2004 to 2006 and 2014 to 2015 outbreaks and the dynamics previously described on incursion years versus expansion years, the 2020 outbreak was expected to begin with new cases in all the same states where last observed in 2019 and then expand outward from those saturated regions. It began as predicted with the first cases of 2020 identified early in the season and in previously affected areas in the lower southwestern states before expanding northward, apparently mirroring expected temporal peaks of vector abundance. However, the expected cases in the Rocky Mountain states (Colorado, Utah, and Wyoming) were never observed. This region, with the most cases in 2019, had zero cases confirmed in 2020 despite strong surveillance and testing. It is known that this outcome is not due to an immunity of the previously exposed animals to the virus. High antibody titers to VSV from previous outbreak years have failed to prevent individual animals from developing lesions in the next outbreak year. Anecdotally, horse owners in historically affected VS-regions have reported that the same horse or horses in their herd developed lesions during every outbreak experienced since living there. In addition, several animals in each outbreak are typically identified presenting with new lesions after the previous lesions have healed on premises where the vector control is determined to have been inadequate. These cases suggest no resistance to infected vector re-exposure with the same virus, despite very high antibody titers, and necessitate the premises be re-quarantined and a more aggressive vector control program administered. There were five such cases documented during the 2019 to 2020 outbreak.

One hypothesis for the 2020 absence of VS cases in the Rocky Mountain region is that the environmental conditions in the area did not support the high-volume of black flies and *Culicoides* spp. that were present in 2019. Specifically, Colorado, Utah, and Wyoming were experiencing extreme drought conditions throughout 2020, which may have impacted the vector hatch and overall insect populations. Further in-depth study is planned to evaluate this hypothesis and investigate other potential causes.

Another unexpected outcome in the 2020 outbreak was the development of a new outbreak region in the Kansas/Missouri/Oklahoma/Arkansas area. Although Kansas and Oklahoma each confirmed a single VSV-infected premises in 2019 in counties bordering active VSV-infected states, neither state had previously reported cases in at least the past 50 years. Kansas and Oklahoma were anticipated to identify more cases in 2020 in western portions of the states where 2019 cases were found, but instead, the 2020 outbreak erupted far to the east in both states and spilled over into western Missouri and northwest Arkansas. More study is needed to evaluate how the virus moved and flourished further east than expected.

Finally, there was a new 2020 incursion of a VSNJV serotype virus in south Texas during the ongoing VSIV outbreak occurring in the western part of the state hundreds of miles away, which is a rare dynamic last observed in the 1997 to 1998 outbreak and has never been fully explained. It is unknown what, if any, VS cases were occurring on the other side of the border in Mexico at the same time, which could provide better insight to the situation. Full genomic sequencing and phylogenetic analysis are planned to investigate the potential origin of both viruses and the relationship of the 2019 and 2020 isolates to viruses circulating more recently in Mexico. All of these unusual occurrences during the 2019 and 2020 outbreaks may be indicators of changes in climatic and environmental factors inducing a noticeable shift in the epidemiology of a historically-observed vector-borne disease.

SUMMARY

VS is a vector-borne livestock disease caused by VSNJV or VSIV. The disease circulates endemically in northern South America, Central America, and Mexico and only occasionally causes outbreaks in the United States. Veterinarians are required to report suspected cases to state and federal animal health officials. Over the past 20 years, VS outbreaks in the southwestern and Rocky Mountain regions occurred periodically with incursion years followed by virus overwintering and subsequent expansion outbreak years. Regulatory response by animal health officials aims to prevent the spread of disease by animals with lesions and manages trade impacts. Equine practitioners play a significant role during VS outbreaks through initial identification and reporting of cases, diagnostic sample collection and submission, management of affected animals, assisting in premises quarantine count-downs and releases, and advising equine owners on biosecurity and vector mitigation procedures. VSV is a zoonotic pathogen that can be transmitted to humans through direct contact with animals that have lesions. Personal protective equipment and good biosecurity practices should be used by veterinarians and animal handlers when handling all animals with active VS lesions. Recent US outbreaks of VS highlight potential climate change impacts on insect vectors or other transmission-related variables, which may result in shifting epidemiology of the disease in future outbreak years.

CLINICS CARE POINTS

- Vesicular stomatitis (VS) is a disease reportable to state and federal animal health officials in the United States. Veterinarians suspecting VS in a clinical animal should contact either the State Veterinarian or the federal Area Veterinarian in Charge (AVIC) for the state in which the animal is located.

- Diagnostic samples to collect in suspect VS cases include a serum sample and swabs of the lesions in viral transport media. Samples must be submitted to a United States Department of Agriculture (USDA)-approved vesicular stomatitis virus (VSV) laboratory with the authorization of the State Veterinarian or federal AVIC.

- VS is a self-limiting disease and the lesions in most affected horses and other livestock heal within a couple of weeks without veterinary intervention; however, some older animals, or those with underlying health conditions, may require supportive care, especially in cases with severe oral lesions where the animals cease to eat or drink.

- Isolation of affected animals and implementation of aggressive vector control measures is imperative to reduce spread of VSV during an outbreak.

- VSV is a zoonotic pathogen that can be transmitted to humans through direct contact with animals with lesions. Personal protective equipment and good biosecurity practices should be used by veterinarians and animal handlers when handling livestock with active VS lesions.

DISCLOSURE

The author has nothing to disclose.

REFERENCES

1. Rodríguez LL. Emergence and Re-Emergence of Vesicular Stomatitis in the United States. Virus Res 2002;85:211–9.
2. Vesicular Stomatitis Outbreak Situation Reports on USDA-APHIS. Available at: https://www.aphis.usda.gov/aphis/ourfocus/animalhealth/animal-disease-information/cattle-disease-information/vesicular-stomatitis-info. Accessed on 11 June 2022.
3. Pelzel-McCluskey AM. Vesicular Stomatitis. In: Winter AL, editor. Merck veterinary manual. online edition. Kenilworth, NJ, USA: Merck & Co, Inc.; 2020. Available at: https://www.merckvetmanual.com/generalized-conditions/vesicular-stomatitis/vesicular-stomatitis-in-large-animals. Accessed on 11 June 2022.
4. Duarte PC, Morley PS, Traub-Dargatz JL, et al. Factors Associated with Vesicular Stomatitis in Animals in the Western United States. J Am Vet Med Assoc 2008;232:249–56.
5. Mohler JR. Vesicular stomatitis of horses and cattle; bulletin No 662. Washington, DC, USA: United States Department of Agriculture; 1918.
6. Hanson RP. The natural history of vesicular stomatitis. Bacteriol Rev 1952;16:179–204.
7. Schmidtmann ET, Tabachnick WJ, Hunt GJ, et al. 1995 Epizootic of Vesicular Stomatitis (New Jersey Serotype) in the Western United States: An Entomologic Perspective. J Med Entomol 1999;36:1–7.
8. Tesh RB, Boshell SJ, Modi GB, et al. Natural infection of humans, animals, and phlebotomine sand flies with the alagoas serotype of vesicular stomatitis virus in Colombia. Am J Trop Med Hyg 1987;36:653–61.
9. Schnitzlein W, Reichmann M. Characterization of New Jersey vesicular stomatitis virus isolates from horses and black flies during the 1982 outbreak in Colorado. Virology 1985;142:426–31.

10. Elias E, McVey DS, Peters D, et al. contributions of hydrology to vesicular stomatitis virus emergence in the Western USA. Ecosystems 2018;22:416–33.
11. Rainwater-Lovett K, Pauszek SJ, Kelley WN, et al. Molecular epidemiology of vesicular stomatitis new jersey virus from the 2004–2005 us outbreak indicates a common origin with Mexican Strains. J Gen Virol 2007;88:2042–51.
12. Rodriguez LL, Bunch TA, Fraire M, et al. Re-emergence of vesicular stomatitis in the western united states is associated with distinct viral genetic lineages. Virology 2000;271:171–81.
13. Velazquez-Salinas L, Pauszek SJ, Zarate S, et al. Phylogeographic characteristics of vesicular stomatitis new jersey viruses circulating in mexico from 2005 to 2011 and their relationship to epidemics in the United States. Virology 2014; 449:17–24.
14. Mason J, Herrera Saldaña A, Turner WJ. Vesicular stomatitis in Mexico. Proc Annu Meet U S Anim Health Assoc 1976;80:234–53. Miami Beach, FL, USA.
15. Peters DPC, McVey DS, Elias EH, et al. Big data-model integration and AI for vector-borne disease prediction. Ecosphere 2020;11:e03157.
16. Pelzel-McCluskey AM. Economic impacts of vesicular stomatitis outbreaks. Equine Dis Q 2015;24:5.
17. Toms D, Powell M, Redlinger M, et al. Monitoring of four naturally infected horses for vesicular stomatitis antibody. In Proceedings of the annual meeting American association of veterinary laboratory diagnosticians, Greensboro, NC, USA, 20 October 2012. Available at: https://www.aavld.org/assets/2012_AnnualMeeting/Proceedings/97280%20aavld12_progabs.proceeding.book.pdf (Accessed on 28 June 2022).
18. Pelzel-McCluskey AM, Christensen B, Humphreys J, et al. Review of Vesicular Stomatitis in the United States with Focus on 2019 and 2020 Outbreaks. Pathogens 2021;10:993.

Moving?

Make sure your subscription moves with you!

To notify us of your new address, find your **Clinics Account Number** (located on your mailing label above your name), and contact customer service at:

Email: journalscustomerservice-usa@elsevier.com

800-654-2452 (subscribers in the U.S. & Canada)
314-447-8871 (subscribers outside of the U.S. & Canada)

Fax number: 314-447-8029

Elsevier Health Sciences Division
Subscription Customer Service
3251 Riverport Lane
Maryland Heights, MO 63043

*To ensure uninterrupted delivery of your subscription, please notify us at least 4 weeks in advance of move.

ELSEVIER